Chiropractors

Their Stories and the

Institutions Leading the Way

Presented by Dealey Media International

www.DealeyMedia.com

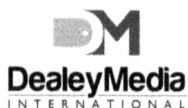

DealeyMedia
I N T E R N A T I O N A L

ISBN-10: 0692573550

ISBN-13: 978-0692573556

www.DealeyMedia.com

This publication is designed to provide general information regarding the subject matter covered. However, laws and practices that often vary from state to state and country to country are subject to change. Because each factual situation is different, specific advice should be tailored to the particular circumstances. For this reason, the reader is advised to consult with an advisor regarding that individual's specific situation.

The author has taken reasonable precautions in the preparation of this book, and believes that the facts presented in this work are accurate as of the date written. However, neither the author nor the publisher assumes any of the responsibility for any errors or omissions. The author specifically disclaims any liability resulting from the use or application of the information contained in this book, and the information is not intended to serve as legal nor medical advice related to individual situations.

Dealey Media International focuses on total market domination for their clients to set them apart in their area and elevate their status as an industry expert and obvious choice for service.

If you are ready to take your practice to the next level, visit our website at www.DealeyMedia.com and register an in depth FREE marketing ASSESSMENT for your business.

ACKNOWLEDGMENTS

We would like to acknowledge those that helped us get this "project of passion" into print and off the ground.

First, to the Dealey Media International team we work with on a daily basis. For months, this project has come up during our weekly project board meetings. You each followed thru with the same DMI "commitment to service" as you do with our clients.

Secondly, to Randy Deavers, Vice President of Operations at Dealey Media International, who spearheaded this project with such enthusiasm. Each time you called or texted after reading a story or when you got thru to a "gatekeeper" was pretty contagious. You never let up. You continued forth explaining "there was no catch" and went on to describe our dream to further the chiropractors that turn the power on in our bodies! You're a gem!

Lastly, a special and heartfelt THANK YOU to Dr. Mike Flynn who caught our passion to further the chiropractic industry by using our major media family ties from over 125 years. The way you opened doors for us was not overlooked and we'd like to say how grateful we are for your effort, and most of all, for your friendship!

Dr. John Carpenter & Niki Dealey

INTRODUCTION

As I look back now, I see the amazing healing power of chiropractic in my life.

Having been in a four car automobile accident twenty years ago, I was left with a bruised spinal chord and a severe lower back injury. My entire right side of my body went "to sleep." I couldn't feel my weight as I could barely walk, I couldn't hold a fork or brush my teeth. Simple every day tasks had to be relearned using my left hand. I was on pretty strong doses of pain killers which remained in my blood stream years later. For a 35 year old woman, active in outdoor activities, this was death to me.

Months and months of therapy and doctor visits were not improving my condition. My doctor basically told me I was most likely not EVER going to feel my left side again.

Growing up I was oblivious to alternative therapies, such as acupuncture, chiropractic, and the like. I became desperate to learn how I could save my quality of life, get off the various medications, and get my life back.

I first started researching chiropractic care. I started there only after seeing more business signs around town of chiropractic clinics than any other alternative medicine therapy.

Imagine my joy, relief, and gratitude, when during a regular medical doctor visit, I could finally feel the pins he was rolling down my left arm, albeit faintly!

Fast forward.......

Life has its curves in the road. About 5 years ago, almost suddenly as I was walking my dog, my knee just gave out. I was not able to place any weight on my left leg and had severe knee pain. I had to skip on my right leg the rest of the way home. After several examinations and second and third opinions, the consensus was that I needed a knee replacement.

I chose to visit several chiropractors, one of which was able to heal me within an eight week time frame. I was able to walk again without assistance. The root cause was due to a gall bladder.

Today, I walk having had no knee replacement. My back pain is completely gone. I take no pain medications, and while by habit, I still eat with my left hand, I can feel my left side of my body!

This book is a labor of LOVE and of DEEP GRATITUDE for those men and women in the chiropractic field. Any chance I get, I urge students contemplating their future career path, to look at the chiropractic path.

Thousands of patients from around the world are served each day by turning the healing power of their own bodies with the precision from very talented and caring doctors of chiropractic, like the ones mentioned in this book.

It is my hope that as you read the stories herein, you are inspired to consider becoming a chiropractor as a profession. There are some amazing chiropractic institutions leading the way from within the industry with cutting edge technologies. This allows their graduates to achieve a higher quality of education that translates to a higher quality of care for their patients.

It is also my hope that you consider whether chiropractic care is right for you after discussing with your primary health care provider.

In closing, proceeds from this book will be distributed to organizations that further chiropractic care and to The Wounded Warrior Project, a charity that is near and dear to me and my husband, Dr. John Carpenter Dealey, who is a HUGE chiropractic fan himself.

> Niki Dealey
> President & Certified Conversion Strategist
> Dealey Media International

Table of Contents

Chiropractors: Their Stories…

Chiropractors:

Their Stories...

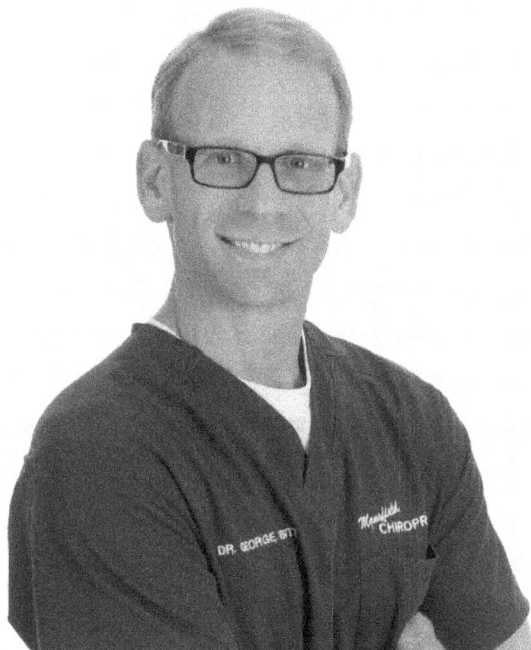

Dr. George H. Bobbitt

"Why and How I Became a Chiropractor"

Growing up I knew I could be whatever I wanted to be. I mostly thought of being a doctor or a lawyer. I was not exactly sure which one, but I knew I liked to help people.

In high school, I made the decision to be a doctor. I enrolled in college at Nicholls State University – known in south Louisiana for its pre-med program. The challenges started early. I married and had a child at the age of 18.

Thanks to my dad, I was blessed to get a job at a local industrial facility to pay expenses. I have tremendous gratitude for my bosses and co-workers who helped me through my college years.

My senior year began with exciting news of being accepted at medical school. Then, I was laid off from my full-time work. I had to go on unemployment, which was not enough to meet our needs. I scrambled to find another job to support my family while I continued with school.

I landed a great job working as a helper for an older man; assisting around his house and with his rental properties. I remember pulling weeds, mowing lawns, pressure washing and helping remodel his properties.

Then, fate moved its huge hand.

As I was cutting my employer's grass, his son approached me to cut his grass too. It turned out the son was a chiropractor with an office nearby. I did not know anything about chiropractic, but because of my interest in health care, I was curious to know more about chiropractic.

As I was preparing to go to medical school, the thought entered my mind to investigate the field of chiropractic. So, I read several books on chiropractic; did more research; and interviewed a couple of chiropractors.

The philosophy and practice of chiropractic resonated with me more than medicine had. In addition, for me to go to medical school, I would have had to relocate my family, find another job and spend another six to eight years on schooling and internships.

In my research of chiropractic, I discovered I could be a doctor of chiropractic in four years as opposed to six to eight for a medical career. I would still have to relocate and find a job, but I wanted to be a doctor as fast as I could to support my family and get my career under way. At this point, I knew chiropractors helped people and that their lives were rewarding.

I made the decision to go to chiropractic school. In 1996, I relocated my family to the Houston, TX area to go to Texas Chiropractic College. I found a job working nights as a supervisor in a chemical plant, and I started chiropractic school that year.

The next four years were a blur of rigorous studies and working hard to support my family. I graduated in 2000 with honors from chiropractic school. I was blessed to land a position as an associate in Bonham, TX with a Dr. Bryan Moore. I relocated my family to this quaint little country town.

I was finally a practicing doctor.

Dr. Moore took me under his wing and helped me get started. However, that first year tested my resolve. Here I was pursuing my dream career, yet I was disappointed with my situation. The practice was not growing and for some reason patients did not like me as the new doctor. They said I was not as good as Dr. Moore. I was working long hours with little mental and financial reward.

Had I made a career mistake? Was being a doctor really my true calling?

Then, I came across an ad that spoke to me. It was one of those "Are you tired of…do you find yourself tired... have you lost your purpose" ads.

I remember signing up to go to the advertised seminar for $49. Dr. Moore advised me not to buy anything and just get the information. The seminar resonated with me and changed my life forever. Its name was "PURPOSE." I embraced the concept and paid for more training. For the first time in my life, I was truly able to see and realize my true purpose. As a result, I helped Dr. Moore triple the practice that year.

It was amazing; my level of certainty and ability to get people well skyrocketed. We built a great practice and helped many people together. I finally realized why chiropractic chose me: to help people get well naturally without the use of drugs or surgery. Chiropractic opened my heart and mind to realize that I had what it takes to make a difference in this world in the field of health care.

After four years of working as an associate, I decided to venture out and open my own practice. I had a desire for a new level of certainty and responsibility. I knew how to be a doctor, but I was not sure how to run a business. So I partnered with a friend, Glenda Davis – now Glenda Tiller, who knew how to run a business and about the administrative aspect of a chiropractic business.

We opened up Mansfield Chiropractic in May of 2004 in Mansfield, TX. It was one of the most exciting and scary times of my life. My family and I moved in with Glenda and her family. Eight of us shared a house and we scrimped by for the first three months of business. We worked 14 to 16-hour days doing whatever was necessary to get ourselves known in the community.

Those long hours, many workshops, many talks and sponsorships paid off. After the first three months, we were paying our bills and starting to collect pay for ourselves. The practice was a success.

Glenda and I started with one staff member for the first three months. By then we had to expand, and after the first year in practice, we added six more team members. Our practice continued to grow and grow. We brought in an associate doctor to help treat the growing number of patients. By the third year in business, we doubled our staff to add more quality to our procedures and patient interaction and treatment.

After three years in practice, we had a desire to help people in a greater way. Sure, we were good at helping people get out of pain, but helping people change their lifestyle and prevent problems from re-occurring was a greater task. We wanted to be more than just a pain relief clinic. We wanted to affect people's lives for long-term better health. Our desire was to help people fix the causes of their problems, not just relieve the symptoms.

This was a bigger challenge than we thought. Most people only go to the doctor when they are in pain. We had to change the way people viewed their health. Our office started to focus on functional issues more than just symptomatic issues. This change in thought process led to our patients to look at their lives differently. Our interest was now to restore function to a body, so that it could do the things it was meant to do.

Through this process, we were able to realize that most people did not understand health and wellness. They thought that as long as they did not have symptoms, they were healthy. However, after a thorough consultation and functional examination they realized that their lives were not as good as they thought.

Once we went beyond just relieving symptoms and began restoring health and function, our practice grew again. We were able to help more people in ways that are more effective and were able to help establish a better quality of life for our patients.

In 2013, we expanded our vision to include helping mentor future chiropractors. Mansfield Chiropractic joined Parker University as adjunct staff in their intern rotation program. This program allows chiropractic interns to learn the art of helping patients get well and the art of running a business at the same time. This experience empowers the interns and gives them real world and real-time experience. We are delighted that our interns have blessed us as much as we have blessed them.

During this time, we decided to expand our territory to help more people through chiropractic. We hired another associate to free me up to concentrate on expansion of our philosophy and chiropractic model.

Our vision was to open a second office to help more people get well and stay well. We choose the nearby community of Kennedale, TX to open our second location. We took what we learned from our Mansfield office and incorporated the best ideas and processes for Kennedale, which opened in May of 2014.

I am amazed at the progress we have made. Our vision of helping others with chiropractic and through chiropractic is happening. To know that not only are we helping people get well naturally, we are also helping our profession expand is heartwarming.

As I look back to what has worked and made the biggest impact over these past 15 years in practice, it has always been PURPOSE.

I did not choose chiropractic. It chose me. Every time I attempt to go in a different direction, chiropractic brings me back to the place where I am supposed to be. I always know when I have moved too fast or have fallen off purpose because chiropractic will humble me back toward my purpose.

I am blessed that God chose me to be a chiropractor, and I am blessed that I have been entrusted with this incredible responsibility of helping people get well.

Mansfield Chiropractic Center LLC

1071 Country Club Ste 101

Mansfield, TX 76063

Phone: (817) 453-3999

Fax: (817) 453-3970

www.mansfieldchiropractic.com

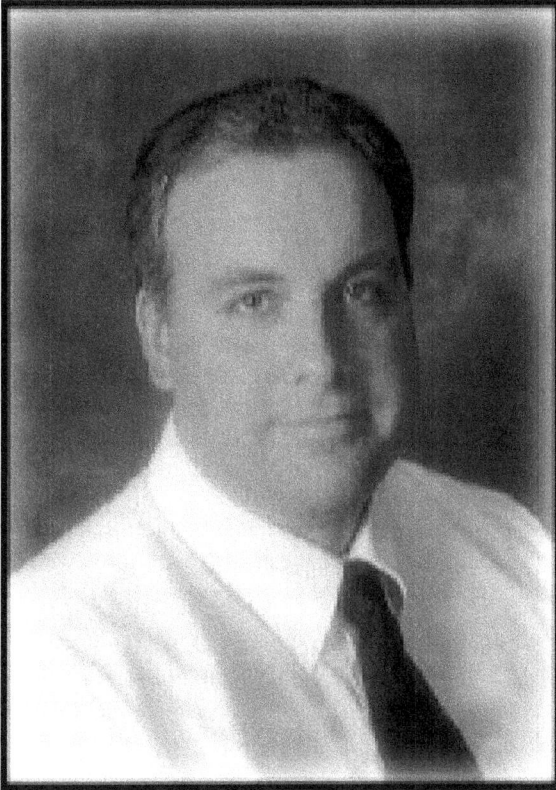

Dr. Matthew R. Roeder

"As a Boy, I Wanted Nothing More..."

As a boy, I wanted nothing more than to be Evil Knievel. If it was daring or dangerous or just plain stupid, I was game: improvising ramps from which to jump my bike or skateboard, jumping off the house, falling from my tree house (once breaking my clavicle with my chin), and falling on my head so many times it became a family joke. I couldn't go fast enough, high enough, or far enough to satisfy the daredevil in me; and if bike helmets and pads existed in the 1960's and '70s, I didn't know about them – and I wouldn't have worn them regardless.

By nine years old I had endured so many traumas, little and big, that my list of symptoms included asthma, chronic muscle spasms in my neck and back, tinnitus, a nervous twitch in my left eye, chronic nasal stuffiness, scoliosis, and a plethora of other difficulties, some of which I didn't even realize weren't "normal" and, as such, had never mentioned to anyone. My parents sought help from a number of medical doctors who scratched their heads, pronounced me "allergic" to practically everything, and suggested that I begin a regular regimen of adrenalin injections. My parents weren't highly educated, and they didn't yet know what the answer would be; but they were wise, and their intuition and common sense told them that injecting their nine year-old son with adrenaline was not the answer.

The answer was presented to my mom while having coffee with a friend. The friend suggested that my parents take me to her chiropractor, Dr. John Whitehead. That single suggestion changed my life.

Dr. John showed us the condition of my spine on X-ray, and explained the source of each symptom, even those I had never mentioned to anyone, including him. He reassured us that if I followed his instructions and received regular chiropractic care, he could help me regain my health and I could be a normal kid, and he was right. After my first chiropractic adjustment, I slept through the entire night without difficulty breathing – something I had not done in years. Over the next few months, my tinnitus cleared, sinuses opened, and muscle spasms relaxed. I felt better than I had in years, and Dr. John was my new hero.

Dr. John talked with me and my parents, and educated us concerning the negative effects my injuries had on my spine and my health in general. We began to understand how the nervous system runs the body, and how misalignments compress and irritate spinal nerves, causing dysfunction in the tissues and organs. I didn't stop all of my daredevil ways; but I did learn to evaluate my choices and understand the consequences, should they not go as planned.

My parents offered to send me to chiropractic college after I graduated from high school; but I chose to go to a trade school instead, because I didn't believe that I could ever be the caliber of doctor that I saw in Dr. John. I became a blue collar worker, suffered many injuries along the way, and continued to benefit from chiropractic care and the close friendships I had with each of my chiropractors through the years.

My mom struggled with cancer much of her adult life, and when I was twenty-nine years old it took her life. I had been searching for an alternate career for several years, and the gifts of healing, strength, and understanding that Dr. John Whitehead gave me were often on my mind. My desire to help others increased as hospice workers came into my parents' home to provide palliative care during my mother's final days, as well as immeasurable comfort that helped us bear up against the pain of our loss.

Mom's passing was, ultimately, the catalyst for my becoming a doctor of chiropractic. I evaluated where I was in life; knowing that drawing a big paycheck but giving very little back was not satisfying my belief that I should help others. My wife, Teresa and I talked and prayed about it, and finally came to the conclusion that the Lord was leading me toward becoming a chiropractor. We sold our home, had a massive garage sale, and took the first steps toward a new life.

Over twenty years later, I sit at my desk in my own chiropractic office, writing my chiropractic story, as I try my best to give my patients the gifts that Dr. John Whitehead gave me so long ago.

Through the years I have had several chiropractic doctors as friends and mentors, to whom I have a debt of gratitude, including Dr. John Whitehead, Dr. Robert Knight, Dr. Steve Kongs, Dr. Dan Waldon, and Dr. Robert Buchanan. Some have passed on, but their care for me will never be forgotten.

The Chiropractic Care Center

2321-A 50th Street

Lubbock, TX 79412

Phone: (806) 793-9005

www.thechirocarecenter.com

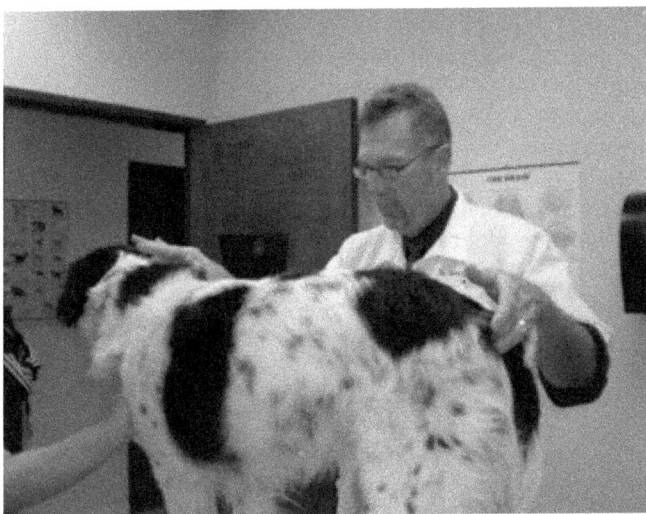

Dr. Gene F. Giggleman, DVM

"My Journey in Chiropractic…"

My journey in Chiropractic started back in 1983. I was a new graduate from Texas A&M College of Veterinary Medicine and had moved to Dallas to join an existing veterinary practice. To supplement my income I took a job teaching Anatomy and Physiology at a local junior college. One evening I received a call from a gentleman telling me he worked for Parker College of Chiropractic and they were looking for teachers. He got my name from the head of the science department at Northlake where I was teaching. I went for an interview to see about teaching at this new Chiropractic College that had recently opened its doors in Irving, a suburb of Dallas. The first question I was asked was if I knew anything about chiropractic to which I responded no, I knew nothing about chiropractic. Then they asked me if I could teach human pathology. Being young and cocky, I responded with, "Give me a book and 24 hours and I can teach anything." The president of the college, a man named Dr. Ted Morter, asked me if I had ever been to a chiropractor. I told him I had not. He took me into his office and began to explain chiropractic to me. For the next 4 hours, that is what we talked about. He explained how the nervous system was the master system of the body and it controlled all other systems and if there was something causing interference to the nervous system all other systems would not work normally. He explained how Chiropractic attempts to determine the root cause of disease, and once that cause is determined, the chiropractor will deliver a chiropractic adjustment, free up the nervous system interference and allow the innate intelligence within the body to reestablish homeostasis and healing could begin. I was fascinated. For the first time I heard someone telling me there is an underlying cause to disease that comes from the body's inability to adapt to stressors and a disruption in the balance of the body (homeostasis). While I was in vet school I had looked into acupuncture and herbal supplements, because even then I was somewhat dissatisfied with what traditional veterinary medicine had to offer our patients. I felt there had to be more, and it appeared I had found what I had been looking for. So I took the job and began a journey that has lasted 32 years.

As I taught classes in this new college, I saw many human patients being treated with chiropractic care and I saw them getting well. Many had suffered for years with existing conditions with no real relief by traditional western medicine and now with chiropractic care they had pain relief and resolution of their clinical conditions.

It made sense to me if this chiropractic works on humans, why couldn't it work on my animal patients? I sought ways to get training in animal chiropractic care but was unable to find classes so being a faculty member at the college I took human adjusting classes and extrapolated it back to my animals. Somewhere around 1992, I got my first opportunity to adjust an animal. A lady with a cocker spaniel called me and told me she was seeking chiropractic care for her dog who had a severe seizure disorder and if we were not able to help the dog she would have to have him put to sleep. My first chiropractic case was a life or death situation, no pressure or anything. I told her to bring him in and let me examine him. When he walked into my clinic, the first thing I noticed was his gait. He was very stiff in the front limbs and hardly moved his neck at all. I reached down to pet him and when I did he fell on his side and started trembling all over. The owner told me this was an example of the seizures he was having. Well I had been out of school about 9 years by the time and seen quite a few dogs with seizures and this looked nothing like any seizure I had ever seen. She told me the medications he was on and said none of them seemed to be working. I picked the dog up and placed him on the exam table and started my examination. His neck muscles were as hard as a rock and every time I touched his neck he would stiffen in pain and start shaking all over. Even though I was a newbie at this chiropractic thing, I could definitely feel his first cervical vertebra (called the atlas) was definitely much higher on the right side than on the left. So I figured this dog must be subluxated and he needed an adjustment. I took my newly acquired chiropractic adjusting instrument, called an Activator ® instrument and turned it up to maximum force, placed it on his atlas and delivered the adjustment. This is when things looked like they went from bad to worse. As soon as I adjusted him he collapsed on the table. All four of his legs went out to the side and his chin hit the table with a thud. Well, I thought I had broken his neck or worse. The lady looked at me with a physiognomy of shock, but I kept my cool and told her it was ok, he just reacted to the adjustment, but inside I was deeply concerned. I quickly picked the dog up and set him on the floor. To my joyous amazement he stood, took about 4 steps forward then shook his head and whole body as dogs do when they are wet and shaking off to dry. The lady was amazed and told me he had not done that in years. I told her all dogs do this after a good adjustment which was true because this was the only dog I had ever adjusted and he did it, so all dogs I adjusted did. I told her to take her dog home and to call me the next day to report his progress. I was fully expecting during the night the swelling would set in from the fractured neck bone, put pressure on his spinal cord and he would pass away during his sleep. But as fate would have it this did not happen. She called me the next day and told me her dog was doing amazing. He had no more "seizures" and he was playing with his toys for the first time in many months. She was overjoyed at the response he had. I explained to her that the "seizures" she reported were not typical seizures and my thoughts were that her dog was in such severe pain from the subluxation in his neck that every time someone would touch him he fell on his side and trembled from the pain. I rechecked him several times over the next few months and the "seizures" never returned. We got him off all the drugs he was on and he went on to live a good pain free life. I was truly impressed with what I had done. Not only did I save this dog from euthanasia, but I successfully stopped his pain and gave the owner her beloved dog back. This brought me a tremendous sense of joy. Wow! This thing called chiropractic was pretty darn cool. I then began to adjust all the dogs I saw in my practice and the results I was getting with nothing short of amazing.

Over the years my practice has evolved to where about 90% of the cases I see are chiropractic cases and only 10% are traditional veterinary practice. During the last 23 years I have had a number of clients bring me their companion animals and tell me their veterinarian had recommended surgery and if they could not afford surgery their animal should be put to sleep. They were seeking chiropractic care because they could not afford surgery and could not bear the thought of having to euthanize their beloved pet. We were subsequently able to get their pet out of pain, get them walking again and put quality back in their life. To know how to treat diseases and reestablish hope, with a relatively inexpensive procedure (surgery can cost thousands of dollars with no guarantee of success) is a blessing second to none.

In 2002 a colleague of mine and I decided we needed to share our knowledge of chiropractic with the world , so with the support and help of Parker College of Chiropractic we started a post graduate program, training veterinarians and chiropractors how to adjust animals. To date, we have trained over 400 doctors to perform chiropractic care on horses, dogs, cats, cows, pigs, birds, raccoons, pet rodents and even snakes. Many veterinarians are unaware of the benefits of chiropractic care and many have preconceived notions about what chiropractic care is so they may be hesitant to refer their patients to an individual trained in animal chiropractic. There is an organization trying to change the negative stigma some have toward chiropractic care. It is called the American Veterinary Chiropractic Association and they have over 600 members all over the United States. I am past president of this organization and graduates of the Parker University animal chiropractic program are eligible to sit for their certification examination.

I would never have dreamed when people would ask me as a kid what I wanted to do when I grew up that my destiny was to teach at a chiropractic school, be the director of a world renown animal chiropractic program, speak all over the United States on animal chiropractic, run a successful animal chiropractic practice and to have published numerous articles on animal chiropractic. All because I answered the phone one night and ventured out to interview for a teaching job in a profession I knew nothing about. It is incredible to me how God works in our lives and I am eternally blessed He chose me to do this.

Parker University Animal Chiropractic Wellness Clinic

2540 Walnut Hill Lane

Dallas, TX 75229

Phone: (214) 902-3456

E-Mail: ggiggleman@parker.edu

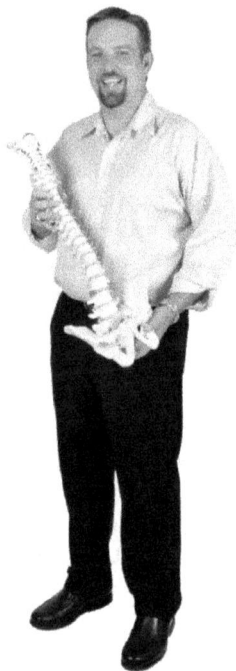

Dr. Steven Brooks, D.C. ACP

"My Path to Chiropractic..."

My name is Steven Brooks and I am a Doctor of Chiropractic. My path to chiropractic school is an interesting tale. I am a first generation Chiropractor and a first in my family to attend college of any type. My father worked in the oilfield of west Texas and my mother was a housewife. My beginnings in chiropractic started at the age of 4 when as a child I had such severe allergies I could not go outside and play with my friends. Fresh cut grass would cause my eyes to swell and nose to run constantly. My mother did the typical pediatrician route and the issue still continued and she was urged to just wait and I would eventually grow out of it. At a friend's suggestion she took me to a chiropractor and after a few treatments my allergies where under control. Growing up I played sports and would find myself back in the office of my chiropractor and as a kid I was always inquisitive. I would watch patients walk in with grimaces and antalgic leans or walks and leave with a smile on their face and a pep in their step. At this point I knew that was for me, I had the calling to serve and help others like my chiropractor had done for me. I researched Chiropractic colleges and soon found that Texas had two colleges, so my search was narrowed. I came to the campus of Parker College of Chiropractic for a tour and was sold instantly that this was the place for me. The founder of the college, Dr. James Parker greeted us and shared his story and vision for Chiropractic. Though he was a small man in stature, his speaking and persona carried him like a giant. I instantly felt the love on the campus and knew again I was choosing the right career and I was in the right place for it. I applied the next day for admission and was accepted shortly after. I attended and graduated Parker College of Chiropractic (now Parker University) and opened my own clinic in 2000. I have a family style practice where I work on newborn babies just hours old to professional athletes to the most senior of citizens. It is amazing to be in practice and see folks with the same issue I had growing up, and it's a blessing to have young adults who choose to be chiropractors because of the service I have provided them. Chiropractic was founded in 1895 by DD Palmer. Dr. Palmer's first adjustment was to Harvey Lillard and it was for deafness. After a few treatments Harvey's hearing returned and the very first Chiropractic success story was born. I am humbled to have my own success stories. Ranging from restoration of hearing just like DD's and Harvey's, to allergy relief like mine, to professional athletes who thought their careers were over only to receive care and go out and set personal records. The daily results of

Chiropractic treatments have endless possibilities for success. I have been honored to be president of the Parker University Alumni association and have served on the board of Trustees. One of my favorite events are speaking to the new class of students about becoming a Doctor and being a successful Chiropractor and then seeing them again at graduation and getting the privilege of leading them in their Graduation oath. Chiropractic is an amazing career and it's a joy to wake up each morning knowing today I get to help folks that need me. My daily rewards come in the form of smiles and hugs from my patients. The ability to help my fellow man in achieving their maximum potential in their performance is a great feeling. I love my profession and my alma mater so much my youngest child was named Parker. I count my blessing daily that I am honored to do what I love and get to share my skills with my patients and colleagues. Being a Chiropractor and having the ability to help so many folks is one of the most rewarding careers that I can imagine. If you are considering a career in Chiropractic I urge you to go tour an office. Follow a doctor around for a few hours and the smiles I saw as a young adult will be the same ones you see today. You will know within a few short minutes in an office if that is your calling. Tour the Chiropractic Schools. Again you will get the sense if that campus is the one for you, much like I did when I met Dr. Parker. Our body's natural instinct is more powerful than most think. When you are in the right place at the right time your body knows. If helping people sounds like a great career, then I urge you to consider being a Doctor of Chiropractic.

Sunset Chiropractic

4116 Sunset Dr.

San Angelo, TX 76904

Phone: (325) 223-5555

www.sunsetchiropractic.net

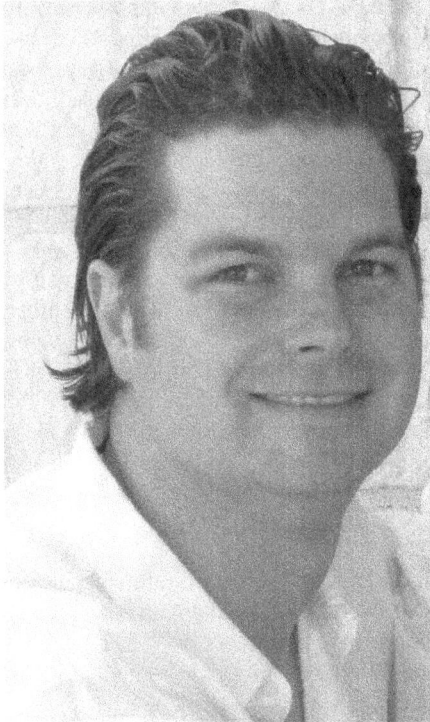

Dr. Chae Tracy, D.C.

"The Power that Made the Body..."

I grew up in a small Oklahoma town and was very active in sports and the outdoors. While always being interested in helping and working with others I decided to pursue a career in a health related field. I discovered chiropractic as a child for various sports related injuries with great results. So my first exposure to Chiropractic was more of an accident and injury standpoint. It took years before I became aware of what Chiropractic truly is and means. Coming from a family history of nurses and pharmacists I decided that a more natural approach to healthcare was of my interest. It was not until a friend and chiropractic student introduced him once again to chiropractic and the possibility of pursuing it as a career. One single thought resonated with me, "The power that made the body heals the body".

At this point I was very excited about where the profession was going and the people's lives that had been changed by chiropractic. After interviewing a multitude of chiropractors, each saying if they had to do it again, they would, without a doubt. At this point I knew that this was the path that God had chosen for him in order to help people. I therefore applied to Parker College of Chiropractic and was awarded a scholarship to attend, and the rest they say is history.

During my first trimester I met my future wife and partner in chiropractic, Dr. Monya. After graduating and receiving The Outstanding Student Achievement Award in 2004, I married my life partner and fellow classmate, Dr. Monya. After traveling Europe and deciding where to begin our lives together we moved to Austin, Texas to begin an eight-month internship.

It was then time to return to a smaller town and begin practicing and sharing chiropractic with others in Dripping Springs, Texas. My primary focus is family wellness with an emphasis on specific correction of the atlas and the body's proper posture.

Some feel that they choose a profession, I feel that Chiropractic chose me and I could not be happier for the fact that it did. Most people get up in the morning and have to go to work. However, I feel that I get to go play. Nothing is more fun for me to see patients getting off of medications and placing them in our drug jug because they don't need them anymore. Kids growing and developing naturally without the aid of drugs, shots, surgeries and sickness. "As the twig is bent so is the tree," shows why it is so important to check children at such a young age. I am the proud father of two girls, Sarys and Ciely. Sarys was a homebirth. It was very clear, maybe too clear, as to the trauma that a child goes through during the birthing process not to mention the nine months prior while in the womb. After witnessing and being a part of such an amazing, natural process I felt compelled to check here little spine. Why? What are we looking for? When the bones (vertebrae) in spine are misaligned putting pressure on the tiny yet delicate nerves that exit at each level then they are not able to innervate the organs properly. In turn this leads to dysfunction which leads to symptoms which leads to disease. As a child their bones are so small and the muscles are so supple that it does not take much to adjust their spine back into proper position with very little force. How much force you ask? It's like sticking your finger into a fresh, warm muffin. However what a profound affect having a proper aligned spine is for a child; that each and every organ and system is growing and developing with 100% innate expression from the brain to the body and the body back to the brain. You see that these children develop the way God intended them to without outside intervention and allowing their bodies to fully express there innate healing and growth potential. To this day, now at age six, Sarys has not had any medications, nor shots and is rarely sick. When she is sick her immune system is compromised, so she gets adjusted and rest and allows the body to heal from above down inside and out. It has been my observation that she gets sick less than her classmates and when ill she recovers quicker than her classmates. Why you ask? She gets adjusted on a regular basis which allows the body to heal and express its full potential in all aspects of life. Your body is able to function at 40%, 60% and up to 100%. The question is where do you want to live life? For the answer is simple, 100%. I get adjusted on a regular basis, every Monday morning. Not because I hurt or have pain or am sick but because I know what it is like to function, keep my brain connect to my body and allow for my Central Nervous System to work and express itself at 100%. When I am subluxation free my focus is clear my energy is at peak levels and my performance is at optimum capabilities. This reminds me of a story about the Gallaher family. "As you know my kids were not excited about someone adjusting them. Now they cannot wait to get their adjustment, as they feel better and are living a healthier life. How many kids do you know that remind their parents of their doctors appointment, so they don't miss it! Your advice and adjustments during my fifth pregnancy made for my best birth yet. Even my newborn baby is in a better disposition after her visit and adjustment each week. Thank you for being people who really care about others and the quality of life they live."

Most folks first seek chiropractic care as a last resort or a first as they don't want to take pill or have a surgery. For example, I can remember Dave said that he considers his spine the most important part of his body. Keeping his spine in order has allowed him to work manual labor while walking, lifting and bending. "Chiropractic care is better than taking pills for your aches and pains as they only act as a band aid, covering up the symptoms yet not addressing the problem." You see, Dave is right. Chiropractic treats the body as a whole not an isolation of individual parts. For example if you wrap a rubber band tightly around your finger what is it going to do? It's going to throb, turn red and start to hurt right? No, we can rub it, take a pill and make it feel better but ultimately have we fixed it? No, we must address the cause, remove the interference. Hippocrates said that when in sickness or in health first look to the spine for answers. And then there are those that seek chiropractic as to avoid drugs or surgery. Let's look at KC for example. Her story begins with having a heart that was beating improperly and her diagnosis was atrial fibrillation, which causes the heart to beat too fast, too slow or with a skipping (irregular) rhythm, better known as arrhythmia. KC learned how the bone (vertebrae) in the upper part of the spine (thoracic) exit the spine to innervate the heart and lungs. Upon examination and x-ray analysis she found that she was indeed subluxated in her cervical spine (neck) and thoracic spine. In fact the exact bones that the nerves exit to innervate (supply) the heart the input it needs to function properly. After the first adjustment her heart started beating more regularly with fewer fibrillations and she started feeling better. Prior to seeking chiropractic care she had planned to have an ablation procedure that would stop the arrhythmia and prevent a future of possible strokes. Armed with knowledge of how the body functions and what controls the nerves to the heart she made the obvious decision to cancel the surgery and start chiropractic care. You see, chiropractic care is not just for aches and pains.

Within chiropractic there are literally hundreds of techniques. Some may be more general and aggressive and others more specific and low force in nature. For example we use a technique called Grostic which means we take very specific x rays and then use an instrument with a low force and very specific adjustment to correct a subluxated atlas. The atlas being the top bone of the spine, and in my opinion, the most important bone in the spine. I will share two stories of the atlas and how people respond when there atlas is properly aligned. Lydia had been getting adjusted on a wellness basis, in her case every other week to maintain her overall health and allow her body to function at 100%. She was very good at recognizing when her atlas was in and when it was out (subluxated.) After a couple of years as I ask her one day as to how she knew and she said to me "I know when my atlas is subluxated because my vision changes and I need to put my glasses on until I get adjusted". Wow, how cool is that? It is not a matter of giving her the magical vision adjustment but rather removing the interference in her nervous system that allows her body to function, and in her case allow her vision to function properly. There are many types of atlas adjustments, this is the one that we specialize in not to say that it is better or superior but as a result we do see phenomenal results.

"My initial reason for in seeking chiropractic care was to support my overall health and wellbeing. In my profession as a massage therapist I am very physical. By receiving adjustments for any subluxations that may present, I know my entire body is receiving optimal nerve conduction to support all my systems. The difference I experience is; increase of energy, clarity of mind, enjoyment being in my body ad decrease of pain or discomfort. The advice I give is to open yourself to greater overall health and wellbeing, mentally, emotionally and physically through natural health care." Sharon S. You see chiropractic is much more then my neck hurt and back hurts. It is about allowing your body to heal and function properly. Cause vs effect? As a chiropractor, most folks come in as a result of the effect however it is important to address and make the patient aware of the effect so as to not continue causing the same problem. Pam F. says, "My reason for starting chiropractic care was because my feet and legs hurt so bad by the end of the day that I literally went home and sat down-no exercise, no fun. I thought I had what I considered a bone spur on my right foot or plantar fasciitis which was extremely painful. Since beginning care I have seen a big difference. The leg and foot pain is almost totally gone and the best part is that I have the added benefit of more energy." Chiropractic treats the body as a whole as opposed to a separation of parts; it would have been easy to just treat Pam's foot. Yet the problem, cause, was coming from the hip and her energy increased as well, the body is not healing and functioning as designed.

If folks knew what we know they would do what we do. That is why these stories must be told. As a county we continue to get sicker and sicker. Heart disease, cancer, diabetes are the leading causes of death in this country. These are lifestyle diseases that cannot be treated with a pill but rather the cause needs to be addressed and then allow the body to heal from the inside, not outside in. "Americans consume nearly 80% of all drugs manufactured in the world. Why then do we rank 37th in overall health in the world?" World Health Organization. This has to change and this message must get out as to how the body heals and what part chiropractic has to do to aide in the healing process. You see, the power that made the body heals the body.

FamilyFirst Chiropractic
(A Total Wellness Center)

800 HWY 290 West Bldg. F Suite 500

Dripping Springs, TX 78620

Phone: (512) 858-WELL (9355)

www.ffchiro.com

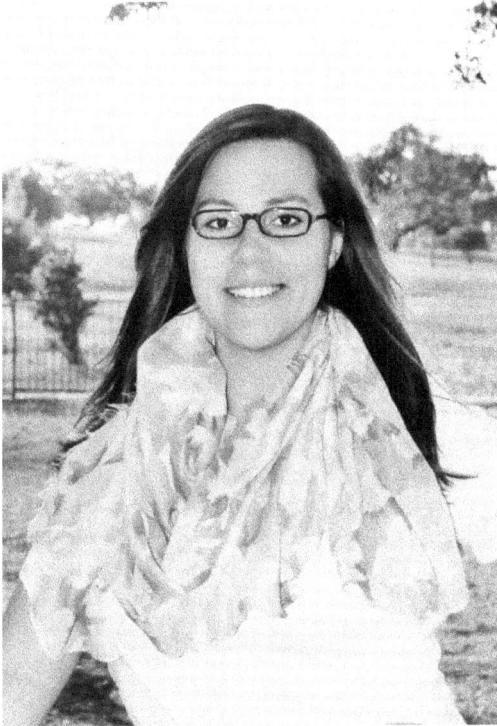

Dr. Annie Wood, D.C.

"Life Happens…"

I am a recent Parker graduate with an established practice in Georgetown, TX. I have faced many struggles and many rewards being a young mom going through school and growing up at the same time. My goals were always to be able to provide financial security for my family but still have the freedom to be involved in my children's lives. With a military husband and three children stability has always been very important. The path I have chosen has lead me to a very different place then I ever imagined.

Life happens and it isn't always in the way we thought it would. I had ambitious goals in high school; I always knew I wanted to be in a profession to help people. Our family physician growing up molded my desire to work in the healthcare industry. My single mother of two struggled and I saw the compassion we were given in our times of need by our family practitioner. I grew up in a very holistic environment where we treated ailments with natural remedies and took care of our body with proper diet and staying active. With an ambition in mind college was a given I just never anticipated my college experience would be so different than most. I fell in love and married my high school sweetheart shortly after he joined the military, we were both 18. As responsibilities changed and we welcomed our first child when we were 19 but quitting college was never an option. With the financial and emotional support of my amazing family and my goal still in mind I continued on in my education. When my husband got back from his first deployment and stationed at Ft. Hood I transferred out of a community college into a University. In my senior year I became pregnant with our second daughter and a decision needed to be made about my goals. It was time to take the MCAT and apply for medical schools. Life's responsibilities started to become a priority before my dreams. It was a conversation with my husband's cousins that changed my whole vision of my future.

I was always treated by Chiropractors growing up; my first encounter was after a car accident where we were rear ended. I thought the doctor was trying to rip my head off! Growing up I always referred to my mom's Chiropractor as her witch doctor. Will and Lana are both Chiropractors and met in school, every family get together they would be treating family. We had many talks about my desire to go to medical school and work with mothers and children. They opened my eyes to world of Chiropractic for pregnancy and pediatrics'. Never did I think my ambition for helping people and my philosophy of health without medication was a possibility. The closest profession was a Doctor of Osteopathy. Since the deadline had come and gone for medical school I researched Chiropractic school. I was surprised how easy it was to qualify and get in since I had been working so hard to be competitive for medical schools. Once I was accepted and set to start in the Fall after graduating from the University of Mary Hardin Baylor with my bachelors I had no idea what my once perfectly planned future was going to look like.

Little did I know that this would be my last summer of freedom and relaxation before I embarked on the new journey I was taking. I enjoyed my kids anticipating our move to Dallas and the new adventure I was about to embark on. My husband was at this point getting out of the military so the kids and I headed out for Dallas while he finished last few months of service at Ft. Hood. It was scary to be starting a new chapter of my life with my two children in a far different place in Texas. When I found out our first trimester consisted of 24 credit hours which was double my normal course load from undergrad I started to worry. I was surprised the size of our class and learning that we would be in the same classroom all day with professor's rotating from room to room. This was much different than what I was use to. I was warned before that Chiropractic school was easy to get in to but hard to stay in. By the end of our first trimester we had lost 15% of our class and we all came out tired and exhausted. It was for sure a culture shock and the beginning of the hardest thing I had ever done. Juggling kids and the course load was no walk in the park. Here I was studying like crazy with 2 small children and making good grades when most students could hardly take care of themselves. People all the time asked me how I did it. My answer would be, "I don't know, I have always been in school with kids and a family, I know nothing else." The balance between family life and school was hard to find. Studying to learn versus studying hard to make A's allowed me to relax and remember I had a family; classes and a degree seemed much easier and obtainable. It was easy to get in the mind set of why I am doing this because the end was so far out of sight. In the beginning people said it goes by fast and gets easier. What they meant was you get use to it and you're always busy so time seems to fly past you.

When the end was finally in sight and we started to get to the classes where we were doing what we came to the school for you could start to see the light in everyone again. With a few scary adjustments under my belt we were thrust into labs where we adjusted each other before we were allowed to touch "real patients". This is where crucial practice came in and some flourished and others struggled. I was shocked that the end was only 3 more trimesters away. My friend Jinna and I went on a Chiropractic mission trip to Haiti where we were able to help 1000's of patients. Our adjusting table was constantly occupied by eager people awaiting the amazing Chiropractic adjustment. We were busy nonstop for 9 hours in the heat each day. It was an experience that reminded me why I was getting into this profession. The physical touch and ability to care for a patient does so much for a person's well being and can impact someone so much. This is why I know all the hard work and stress was worth it. Having a person hug me and thank me for giving them relief from pain and they can dance with their husband again which it has been years because she was unable to. This is what assures me that even though Chiropractic was not my first choice it was my right choice. After the trip I came back fired up to be set free on the public and their spines.

Another turn in my life plans happened right before our clinic started. I became pregnant with our third child, a long awaited son! At this stage in Parker most of my classmates were getting married or having babies. This was a crucial time in our studies to really prepare for the real world and a good representation on what we should expect in building our own practice. Being due right before graduation definitely had me working harder than most to finish our requirements before baby came. I have always been a hard worker and when I set goals I accomplish them. I met hours for each of the 3 trimesters easy, getting patients and our required adjustments was harder. However with an amazing mentor and clinic doctor I learned all the necessary skills to acquire and effectively treat my patients. With no ambition to open up on my own after school I fluffed off in our business building classes. Who needs a business plan or to know how to keep track of stats? I knew I wanted to work for someone and learn from their mistakes before leaving the nest and flying. Graduation came fast and as I looked back on the years at Parker and where all the fresh faced classmates have now blossomed into unrecognizable young doctor's ready to make a difference in the health field.

Things were not what I had expected after graduation. Even though I found a job right away, near home, my high expectations where shortly shot down. I was excited about my job even though I thought I was worth more than the start off pay. I soon got disappointed by the hours I was working and my vision of practicing Chiropractic was not the same as the owner. Looking for another associate position and now knowing what to look for in a place to work it was hard to find a place I would love working in. After a month of finding nothing an idea popped in my head, if I can't join a place that I think I would love working at then I should make my expectation of a practice come true. This was the one little thought that brought me to my current life path. I am now the owner of a thriving practice in Georgetown. Never did I think I would open my own practice nor did I have the desire. Life is funny in working itself out the way it is suppose to be. In the first year not only are we not bankrupt like my husband was expecting, I was voted the best Doctor in Georgetown 2014 and making profit well before expected. I have been blessed in life with a beautiful family and many things to be thankful for. I change people's lives every day and get to witness joy every day. People come into my office in pain and leave with smiles. So it makes sense to have the most perfect name for my vision, Blessed Family Chiropractic.

Blessed Family Chiropractic

101 Cooperative Way Suite 235

Georgetown, TX 78626

Phone: (512) 868-6900

Fax: (512) 868-6995

Email: blessedfamilychiro@gmail.com

www.blessedfamilychiro.com

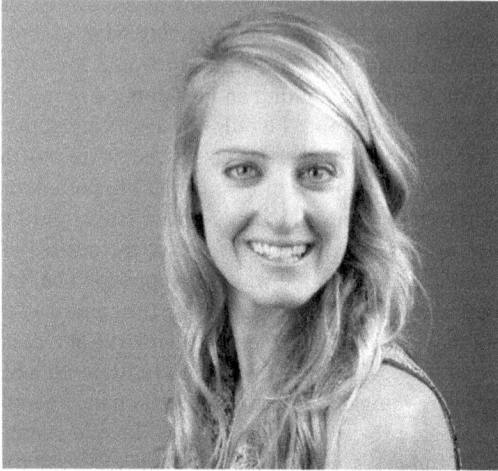

Dr. Sarah Potthoff

D.C., C.K.T.P., F.A.K.T.R.

"Teamwork, Integration, and Collaboration…"

From the beginning, my chiropractic story has been one of teamwork, integration and collaboration – even before I knew these principles they would lay the foundation for my passion and dedication to the profession and society. Everyone I encountered in this story played a vital role. The journey began when I discovered my passion for helping others through healthcare and crystallized when I realized the growing need for non-invasive options for musculoskeletal in American Healthcare.

Initially I thought medical school would be my next step after undergraduate college. I had a passion for helping others and a fascination with human anatomy and physiology. However my perspective changed after talking with medical students and fellows because of the lack of emphasis on prevention of illness. I had seen a chiropractor since I could remember for many ailments and attributed my injury-free high school and division one college career to the chiropractic care. With encouragement from a chiropractic uncle, I decided to shadow female chiropractors in practice (I had always gone to male chiropractors – and was unsure of the techniques and chiropractic care from a female perspective). Shortly after observing and meeting so many empowering women, I enrolled in at Cleveland Chiropractic College in Kansas City.

Ironically enough I always imagined chiropractic care within the confines of modern medicine facilities. I was confused with the disconnect between these two worlds – modern medicine and chiropractic care. As I learned more about the American healthcare history, culture and currently environment I was drawn to the gap for musculoskeletal care and saw myself as a solution. To gain a better understanding of the missing links between these two worlds, I shadowed orthopedic surgeons and primary care physicians . It taught me how to collaborate between the multidisciplinary scopes of practice and kept my passion burning.

This passion fueled my interest to dedicate myself to my studies, emphasizing the most recent evidence based theories and involvement in various chiropractic clubs and in the student body. I pursed and obtained an internship at Walter Reed National Naval Medical Center in Bethesda, Maryland. I provided chiropractic care at the hospital-based chiropractic clinic under the direction of Dr. William Morgan. Second, I was allowed to perform weekly rotations with other departments medical fellows including: Pain

Management, Neurosurgery, Orthopedic Surgery, Radiology, Diabetes Clinic, Physical Medicine and Rehabilitation, Physical Therapy, Occupational Therapy, and Oral Facial Pain Clinic. Third, I also had the opportunity to be the Naval Academy Football Team Chiropractor.

Upon graduation in December 2011 from Cleveland Chiropractic College, I decided to volunteer for the non-profit organization World Spine Care to continue my journey of integrating chiropractic care within the medical model. I chose World Spine Care because of its mission to provide evidence-based integrative prevention, assessment and treatment of spinal disorders and musculoskeletal conditions in developing countries. I gained insight into the Botswana health care system while treating patients at the Mahalapye District Hospital, and discovered clinical and cultural challenges that enlightened my perspective on integrative health care.

Beyond the walls of Mahalapye Hospital, I assisted in the further development, testing, and documentation of World Spine Care protocols. These protocols are implemented in the WSC clinic in Shoshong, a rural village about 35 kilometers outside Mahalapye. The clinic in Shoshong opened in July 2012 and serves as a pilot project for World Spine Care, providing multidisciplinary spinal care services previously unavailable for this population.

After a year in private practice, I had the opportunity to follow my passion for providing chiropractic care within a collaborative, multidisciplinary clinic in Gaithersburg, Maryland called Casey Health Institute. Casey Health Institute (CHI) is truly one of its kind; a non-profit primary care office which is a patient-centered medical home (PCMH). It offers a vast array of complementary and alternative modalities in addition to primary care, which offers the perfect environment for collaboration, integration and teamwork. I continue to enjoy the patient-centered care I provide at CHI, collaborating with other healthcare providers, and integrating chiropractic care into a primary care setting.

Casey Health Institute

800 South Frederick Avenue

Gaithersburg, MD 20877

(301) 664-6464

www.caseyhealth.org

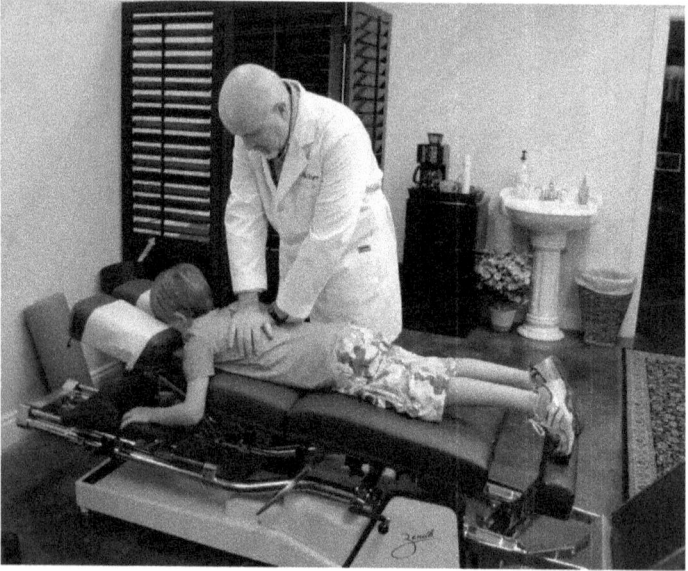

Dr. J. Michael Flynn

D.C., F.I.C.C.

"A Life Well Lived"

My journey to becoming a doctor of chiropractic can be traced back to my grandmother Violet. While her only son Jack (my dad) was serving in the Army during WWII, she experienced neck pain and headaches. When she told her doctor that she could not tolerate the medicine he prescribed for her, she was told that there was nothing else he could do. Fortunately for my grandma, a girlfriend who knew she was suffering, brought her an advertisement from a new kind of doctor - a chiropractor. The ad said he treated headaches without using medication. My grandmother made an appointment and after several visits of upper neck "adjustments," she was pain free.

When my Dad returned to Detroit after the War, his mother encouraged him to consider becoming a chiropractor. He had never heard the word -- much less knew what they did. Dad looked into it by visiting several chiropractors. He liked what he heard and watched in patient care, without drugs, focused on analyzing the structure of the body and making adjustments to the spine and pelvis. He moved with my mom and older brother to Davenport, Iowa where he enrolled at Palmer College of Chiropractic. This is where my sister and I were born. Following an early childhood accident, which put me in the hospital, my parents took me for my first adjustment to Dr. Bartlett Joshua Palmer, then president of the college. He was known as B.J., and was the son of Daniel David Palmer, who is credited with the founding of the chiropractic profession. The word chiropractic is Greek, and translates to "treatment by hand."

Dad graduated with a Doctor of Chiropractic (DC) degree in 1954 and was influenced by Dr. B J to set up his practice in one of the four remaining states that did not yet have regulation for his profession. He chose Louisiana, not realizing it would be the last state to license the profession in 1974. Even with a busy schedule of patients, practicing for 20 years in an unlicensed environment was a hardship for him and his family. Chiropractors in Louisiana were under the constant threat of arrest for practicing medicine, and their professional status in their communities was not accepted by the establishment.

There were always whispers of "quack" and "cultist" associated with the reputation of his new profession. The last two chiropractors to be jailed for practicing chiropractic in the United

States were in Louisiana in January 1975. Although the Louisiana law had been passed in June of 1974, two Shreveport chiropractors, who had been arrested and charged prior to the law, were ordered to prison for several days.

Following my undergraduate education in psychology at the University of Southwestern Louisiana, I chose to follow my father, attending Texas Chiropractic College in Houston for four years. I graduated in 1975 - one year after Louisiana DCs were granted legislative approval and five months after the last chiropractors were sent to jail. My Dad was chosen by the Governor to be on the first board of chiropractic examiners - an important position I would also later serve for eight years. I have a younger brother Victor, who is a graduate of Parker University in Dallas (formerly Parker College of Chiropractic) and has a successful chiropractic practice in New Orleans

One of the "backdrops" to the emergence of chiropractic as a health profession is highlighted by what is known as the Wilk Case. In 1976, Chester Wilk DC and four other doctors of chiropractic sued the American Medical Association (AMA) for violations of the Sherman Antitrust Act. Until 1983, the AMA held that it was unethical for medical doctors to associate with chiropractors and labeled chiropractic, "an unscientific cult." After a lengthy and costly legal battle, the AMA and 1900 local medical societies were found guilty in September of 1987 for violations of the Sherman Act.

The Judge stated in her ruling that the AMA had engaged in an unlawful conspiracy in restraint of trade with the intent, "to contain and eliminate" the chiropractic profession. Among the Judge's findings were that the AMA had a long history of illegal behavior that was successful in damaging the reputation of the chiropractic profession. This prompted her to issue a permanent injunction to prevent such future behavior. The chairman of that "special" AMA committee to eliminate the chiropractic profession was from New Orleans. This might answer any question of why Louisiana was last to license the profession.

Few, if any, other professions have had to endure such a significant and "mean-spirited" challenge to their development. The chiropractic profession stood the test, but their reputation took a "hit."

The history of the chiropractic profession dates back to its beginning in 1895. The first states to license the profession were in the early 1900's and chiropractic grew steadily as a healing art, philosophy and science. Today, there are 18 chiropractic colleges and universities in the United States and near twice that number throughout the world. A minimum of seven years is required to achieve a doctor of chiropractic (DC) degree. This is my ninth year serving on the board of trustees for Parker University.

I am in my fortieth year of a chiropractic practice that my father began. The opportunity to care for patients of all ages is a privilege that I am grateful for every day. It has been a great honor to have served as chairman of the board of the American Chiropractic Association and later president of the World Federation of Chiropractic, which has ninety international country member chiropractic associations. These positions have given my wife and I many occasions to travel to many parts of the United States and around the globe, experiencing different cultures and meeting wonderful people.

Almost every day I see patients who began their chiropractic care with my father. They always have great stories to tell about those early days of my dad's practice. It is with pride that I tell them of the progress of the profession which includes the United States Olympic Committee appointing a chiropractor to be Director of Sports Medicine Clinics. This DC oversees the clinics at the Olympic Training Centers in Colorado, California and New York. He and the USOC sports medicine team are actively involved in building an integrated, multi-disciplinary approach to health care, injury treatment and prevention, and service for US Athletes. The team includes a wide-range of health care professionals including chiropractic and medical physicians. Doctors of Chiropractic can also be found on most professional, college and high school teams, caring for athletes in all sports, while integrating care with other health specialties. This is quality health care.

It is not uncommon to see a patient who will tell me he or she saw a chiropractor while serving in the military. Over a decade ago, Chiropractors received Congressional approval to care for active duty military personnel and also have hospital privileges in the Veteran's Administration (VA) hospital system. In the late 1990s, the Department of Defense (DoD) conducted a study where they placed two chiropractors at 13 military sites including Bethesda Naval Hospital and Walter Reed Military Hospital. Five years later, when the results of the study were revealed, the DoD found that compared to traditional medical care, chiropractic care resulted in higher levels of patient satisfaction, fewer hospital stays, required less medication and achieved significant improvements in military readiness.

For nearly 15 years, doctors of chiropractic have been on staff at the Office of Attending Physicians located in the US Capitol. These doctors, of different specialties, only care for members of Congress and the US Supreme Court. Chiropractors are also being welcomed into the growing trend of on-site corporate clinics and are part of the Affordable Health Care Act, enacted to curb rising cost and provide outcome-driven health care. Chiropractors have been included in the medical-home model of the future and have been part of the Medicare system since 1973.

The chiropractic approach to health care brings a focus to whole body structure and function with an emphasis on movement biomechanics. The philosophy centers on the relationship of the brain and spine to the nervous system. The art is corrective manual adjustments by hand, or in some cases instrument assisted devices, to improve joint motion and effect posture, balance and neurological expression. Advice on nutrition, hydration, stretching, exercise, soft tissue rehabilitation, stress management and healthy lifestyle choices are part of the education and clinical training of chiropractors. Acute and chronic conditions are regularly seen by chiropractors. Consequential conditions as a result of motor vehicle accidents and work related injuries are often found in chiropractic clinics. Children and senior citizens are a large part of most chiropractic practices.

As the public learns more about chiropractic care, and clinical research continues to provide evidence of effectiveness, there will be greater demand and utilization of chiropractic. It is a natural, rational treatment option that for many common conditions says, "Try chiropractic care first, drugs second and surgery as a last resort." The time is near when doctors of chiropractic will be among the most respected members of the health care system - respected for their non-pharmaceutical, conservative, preventative and patient-centered approach.

The quote attributed to the inventor Thomas Edison (1804-1896) is a guide to chiropractic care – "The doctor of the future will give no medication, but will interest patients in the care of the human frame, diet and in the cause and prevention of disease."

Chiropractic has proven to be safe and effective in the care of headaches, neck and back pain. These are among the leading causes of disability and visits to a doctor. As expanded research is undertaken to validate the positive outcomes accomplished with chiropractic care, there will be new discoveries beyond neuro-musculoskeletal care. These discoveries will embrace the relationship of structure and function to human physiology and healthier immune and viscerosomatic systems.

The doctor of chiropractic plays an important role in educating patients. Many of today's patients are overmedicated, undernourished, out of shape, carry too much weight, sit much more than they should and are highly stressed. Patients of the future must acquire a higher set of standards to achieve a healthier and more productive life. The announcement by The Centers for Disease Control and Prevention in 2011 that classifies prescription drug abuse as an epidemic gives reason for patients to consider alternative treatment methods. Chiropractors often recommend acupuncture, massage, yoga and meditation.

In order to achieve a healthier society, patients of the future will have to acquire a better understanding of their personal responsibility for their health. They will learn the importance of the foundations of health based upon good nutrition, hydration, exercise, rest, weight control and stress management. They will think prevention with a goal of a fit life. They will seek non-pharmacological ways to manage their health, when possible. They will seek doctors who counsel and advise their patients on healthy lifestyle choices and the consequences of bad choices.

The patients of the future will visit doctors who care for them with structural adjustments for better functional alignment to improve their posture, joint mobility, and flexibility. These patients will have a better appreciation of their mental and emotional state of being, striving to always have an optimistic attitude, replacing worry with positive expectations. The patient of the future will insist that doctors of all specialties work together for the best outcomes in personal health and well-being. All patients deserve doctors who practice by the bioethics principles of primum non nocere, the Latin phrase that means. "First do no harm."

Many of these patients of the future are being seen today in my clinic and in the clinics of over seventy thousand DC's across the United States. As the legendary poet and author Victor Hugo once said, "Nothing is more powerful than an idea whose time has come."

I will be forever grateful to my grandmother, for among many things being largely responsible for my career. I reflect on how thankful I am for her girlfriend pointing her in the chiropractic direction. Grandma told me that she experienced several episodes of neck pain and headaches in her life. She always saw a chiropractor as soon as she could, and with chiropractic care her symptoms abated. It was a proud moment for me when grandma first asked me to give her an adjustment. Among so many things that my father shared with me was a guiding principle, "to treat every patient like they were a member of your family." Finally, I have to mention my beautiful Scottish mother Pat. My sisters, brothers and I were blessed to be raised in a loving home. Strong in her convictions and loyalties, she was a model of unconditional love in our lives. My three daughters were fortunate to have my mom in their lives, and along with my five grandchildren are blessed to have learned the lesson that a life filled with love is a life well lived.

Holistic Health Medical Center

Flynn Clinic of Chiropractic

567 Corporate Dr.

Houma, LA 70360

Phone: (985) 223-3811

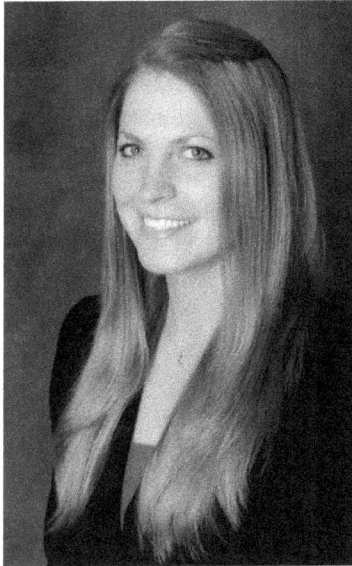

Dr. Stephanie Johnson, D.C.

"Serving my Community"

It all started with dance. At age six, I innocently embarked on my journey into health and wellness with my first ballet class. Unbeknownst to me (or anyone else) my evolution into a chiropractor had begun.

I grew up dancing ballet and switched to modern in college. I graduated from UC Berkeley with degrees in subjects I was most passionate about. I received a Bachelor of Art in Dance Performance Studies and a Bachelor of Science in Nutritional Science/Toxicology. Upon graduating, I was undecided where in the health and wellness industry I wanted to next invest myself. Saddled up with a great education in subject matters I loved, I was well on my way to finding a career of service that resonated with my values and interests.

Dance was the overriding theme that carried me through my undergraduate studies, and fueled my passion for nutrition at Cal. Still fascinated with movement and wellness, I was hungry for more information. For two years after college I continued to make dance a priority. I went through a Pilates teacher training course and picked up distance running. Determined to learn more, I worked as an assistant for a physical therapist, and eventually an assistant for an orthopedic office with five physicians. Tackling everything that interested me, I then went through yoga teacher training, and studied for (and took) the MCAT. I started taking a few classes at the local community college that I still needed as pre-requisites for graduate school. Although I was still undecided what specific degree I wanted to pursue, I knew it would be health-related, and the pre-requisites were essentially universal for those programs.

Knowing that I would go into health and wellness was a no-brainer, but choosing my specific path took time, because I was interested in everything. It was common for me to romanticize careers, and to assume I would resonate with everything I embarked upon. My mission was to fine-tune which career I would connect with most. I was on the hunt to figure out whether I wanted to be a physical therapist, acupuncturist, chiropractor, medical doctor, osteopath specializing in manipulative medicine, or naturopath. I began an interview process and met with several chiropractors, an acupuncturist, two osteopaths (one who specialized in manipulative medicine), and a naturopath.

By this point I had narrowed down my selection to either chiropractic or osteopathy. I had actually never heard of an osteopath until I began my career investigation, and my dad mentioned that my great-grandmother had graduated as an osteopath in 1913. When I first learned of the profession, I became very excited. Osteopathy seemed to be a perfect combination of medicine and chiropractic. I had always been a fan of manipulative care, because as a dancer, I had been under regular chiropractic care since I was 13. I also liked that osteopathy allowed prescription rights. As I continued on my journey to find my calling, two key factors came into play that had a major impact on my career choice.

First, mastering the art of adjusting the human frame was of utmost importance for me. Upon further investigation in osteopathy, I learned that osteopathic schools in the United States nowadays are more comparable medical schools in their curriculum. With their increased focus on surgical and pharmacological interventions (compared to the profession's inception in 1874), time spent teaching manipulative techniques has decreased. Learning how to adjust is a process that requires patience and much practice. I realized I would receive a greater concentration of training in manipulation going to school for chiropractic.

Second, my desire for prescription rights completely flipped upside-down after working for the orthopedists. I learned to admire the great responsibility allopaths and osteopaths take on every time they write a prescription. Many times I encountered patients who tried their best to manipulate the physicians for pain medication. It was disturbing. One instance in particular completely confirmed that I did not want to enter a field that prescribes.

One day while I was on the job with one of the orthopedic surgeons, an individual was seen in the Emergency Room for a horrible infection in his leg. This person recreationally used illegal narcotics, had accidentally sliced his quadriceps with a hatchet one day, had sewn it together himself with dental floss, and inevitably developed an infection. Here began the search for a prescribed painkiller that faced three challenges. One, the medication needed to not have an adverse reaction to his recreational drug use. Two, it needed to not be so addictive that the patient would become dependent. And three, the medication needed to be strong enough that the patient would not be inclined to increase recreational drug use. This, obviously, became a phone call to the pharmacologist for guidance. The event opened my eyes even more to the challenges and responsibilities of prescribing: from allergies and adverse reactions, to improperly prescribed drugs and unknown drug interactions, to dependency. While I commend those who regularly juggled this constant challenge, I lost interest in wanting the ability to prescribe.

During my time working with orthopedic surgeons, I gained the insight I was hoping for regarding how I resonated with the profession. When it came to trauma, fractures, surgeries, and emergency situations, these individuals were incredible. They have saved lives and improved outcomes of horrible accidents immeasurably. But I also recognized that this was not my passion for a career path. I craved to work with the sizable demographic of patients who were not trauma cases and who were not candidates for surgery or injections. For these patients, I found the tools left in the allopathic toolbox limiting. These patients were given a diagnosis (usually following an x-ray), possibly a prescription for pain medication, and a referral to a physical therapist to rehab the pain they were experiencing. Sometimes this worked remarkably. Other times these patients would come in again a month later, and the cycle would repeat itself. It would become frustrating for the medical doctors because they wanted to help, but were limited with what they personally had to offer these patients.

My experience working with medical doctors helped to fine-tune how I wanted to serve as a health professional. I wanted to serve the demographic that represented the huge grey area of pain and malaise where drugs, injections, and surgeries were not reasonable solutions because "nothing was wrong." I wanted to work with my hands and be a master at a kinesthetic trade. I wanted to focus on movement and improving quality of life. I wanted to have the education to differentially diagnose musculoskeletal problems from other more serious issues that warranted a referral to a primary care physician or orthopedist. Not only did I want to be able to diagnose a musculoskeletal problem, but I wanted to be able to personally be a part of the solution through manual care, education, and prevention.

I took a step back and asked myself what profession I truly wanted to pursue. I wanted to be a chiropractor. It was clear after all my education in the classroom and in the field, that chiropractic was the career of service that resonated with my values and interests most.

Palmer College of Chiropractic West became my alma mater several years later. Shortly before graduation, I moved from California to Washington DC for an opportunity to complete my clinical internship at the Walter Reed National Military Medical Center, where I worked with wounded veterans coming home from the Middle East. Upon graduation, I decided to stay in the DC area. It was the drive of the people in the region, and the plethora of opportunities to grow in my field and connect with other like-minded medical professionals, that influenced my decision to stay on the East Coast.

I currently practice as an independent contractor in Annandale, Virginia. There is no doubt in my mind that I am living my dream job. The education and skills I have acquired have allowed me to help others in ways that warm my heart and serve others well. I am able to spend time with my patients and provide thorough care. My schedule allows me to go trail running weekly with my colleague at lunch, go salsa and swing dancing in the evenings, and to continue teaching and practicing yoga. I make sure to get adjusted at least once per week. It behooves all health professionals to model the quality of life they are promoting to their patients. I live and breathe health and wellness, and strive to live by my daily mantra: "If your doctor isn't the healthiest person you know, find another doctor," (source unknown). I am a chiropractor through and through and I love what I do. Chiropractic is who I am, who I always have been, and how I best serve my community.

Positively Chiropractic

5105-A Backlick Road, Annandale, VA 22003

Phone: (703) 642-8685

www.posichiro.com

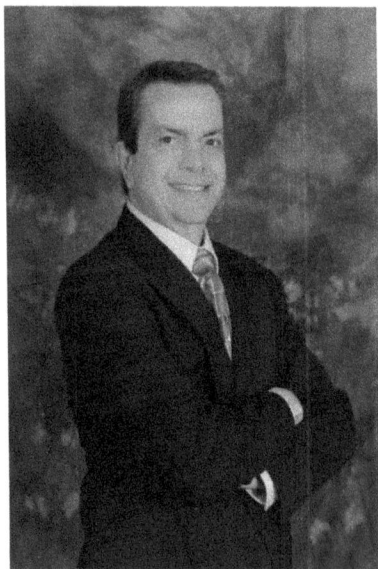

Dr. Louis D'Amico, D.C., R.Ph

"My Career in Chiropractic..."

My career in chiropractic has allowed me to travel around the United States and around the world meeting and training chiropractors from many different countries. I am always interested in hearing how each of them found chiropractic. In most instances it was because a prior chiropractor and/or chiropractic care had a profound impact on their lives. Most often it was because chiropractic care was able to resolve a condition or conditions that were not adequately helped by conventional orthodox medicine. Many times these individuals were left with little hope that they would ever be able to overcome the particular affliction that had affected them. That prior chiropractic care gave them their lives back and for that they decided to become a chiropractor so they could help others. Chiropractors are some of the most compassionate and service oriented individuals that I have ever met. The following is my story.

My name is Dr. Louis D'Amico and I grew up near Pittsburgh, Pennsylvania. I was born in 1956 and my parents never graduated high school. My father went into the steel mill at age 16 to help the family and then got drafted into World War II when he was 19 years old. He married my mother and went off to war. When he returned he continued his tenure in the steel mills and spent 43 years there. Like many in that greatest generation that ever lived he went to work every day in very dirty and dangerous conditions to hopefully provide a better life for his family. Many times I had the opportunity to work summers in the steel mill with really good pay compared to the minimum wage but he would not let me do it. He told me that he wanted me to go to college so that I never had to work in that "sweat house". Most of my aunts and uncles as well as my friends during those times had similar lifestyles as the steel mills and their ancillary businesses were growing dramatically and jobs were plentiful for anyone who wanted to work.

I always loved math and science in high school, and in 1979, at the age of 22, I graduated Magna Cum Laude from the West Virginia University School of Pharmacy. I planned to work a few years, get some good experience, save up some money, and then eventually move on into medical or dental school. In other words, pharmacy was going to be a steppingstone toward something bigger.

At the blink of an eye a decade went by and during those 10 to 12 years I enjoyed a very decent income, was single, and did a lot of traveling. But something woke up inside me and said you're not getting any younger so it's time to move on to those bigger goals if you're going to do it. So I took a Medical College Admission Test review course and then took the exam. The counselor told me that with my current degree, past work experience, and test scores I could get into most medical schools except for maybe Ivy League schools. The University of Pittsburgh Medical School was only 20 miles away from me so I decided that I would apply there. I can remember being on campus in Scaife Hall to pick up my admissions packet. I sat and watched all these very hurried young medical students rushing around here and there. I started to do the math as I would have been 32 when I entered medical school and then added on the four years to complete an anesthesiology residency and thought oh my god I'll be over 40 years old by the time I get out. So I never turned in the application.

For some gut feeling reason, medical school was just not feeling right, so I spent some time investigating dental school as the University of Pittsburgh has a very good dental school nearby as well. I talked with my dentist and a few of his colleagues but again no burning desire to invest that time of money into dental school was there. It was during these years that I began to develop a slow and insidious onset of right-sided cervicothoracic pain and tension headaches. At first they were barely noticeable but over time they became more frequent. It always seemed like I was rubbing my neck or had to take something like ibuprofen at the end of the day for the headache. I was working retail pharmacy at the time and these were 12 hour shifts where we would manually fill 200 to 300 prescriptions a day. Please remember that this was before computers, so we were typing labels by hand as well as counting and pouring all the various pharmaceutical drugs. We were also responsible for managing the full store so the job could become quite stressful at times. I did not realize the cumulative stress that was building in my neck but can tell you that I was very annoyed with it.

It was during that time that I began to date a girl who eventually became my wife. Her name is Angi. I would come off of a 12 hour workday and ask her to please rub the knots out of my neck and upper back. She was always amazed how tight and ropey these muscles had become. Every time she would rub my neck she told me that I needed to see her chiropractor. This was around 1991. I had seen chiropractor signs along the road but never knew what they did. I had been in such good health that I was rarely at the medical doctor during those years. Except for a physical every one to two years I was in great shape. I never really had any prior significant injury to my neck or back as well. And of course, all of my training as a pharmacist was done in very modern hospitals and clinics.

A few months prior to dating Angi I made an appointment for my neck at a reputable orthopedic group, had an exam and cervical x-rays, was told that there was nothing wrong, that it was stress and tension, and they gave me pain pills to use when needed. Since I was a pharmacist, this all made perfect sense.

I asked Angi why she had seen a chiropractor and she told me that she had a prior neck injury which caused headaches and she was eating aspirin like candy. She went to the hospital and also her medical doctor and they told her to just keep taking the pain pills. A friend referred her to a chiropractor and the relief was almost immediate and that she was not having many headaches or neck pains anymore. I told her that I had visited a "real doctor" before dating her and they told me nothing was wrong. Her argument was if there was nothing wrong then why was I still having all this neck pain and headaches? So I decided to follow her device and have a chiropractic evaluation. Now her chiropractor was very old school. This practice was in an old house and the decor was out of the 1950s and 60s. When I pulled up to the office that first day I really thought I should just keep driving on. But ever so skeptical I went in and filled out the paperwork. The doctor looked at my x-rays and listened to my story and then began to palpate my neck and upper back. During this time he began to explain innate intelligence and the body's natural ability to heal itself. He explained that my job as a pharmacist required prolonged standing with the telephone in my right ear keeping it there with my hunched up right shoulder while I used my hands to type, count, and pour. He told me that his adjustments would reduce nerve interference in the joints of my neck and upper back which would then calm down the tight muscles and reduce the frequency of the headaches as well as restore my normal cervical range of motion. Everything he said resonated with me but I was still very skeptical. After a few sessions at his office, however, I began to feel noticeably better and everything that he predicted would happen eventually did. He also gave me stretches to do regularly to reduce the tension of my head and shoulders pulling on my neck and upper back while at work.

Over time this doctor and I became friends and over lunch or dinner we would discuss this thing called chiropractic. He sent me to the public library to read a few books about the profession which I did and over the next few months I became more and more interested in the concept of natural healing versus the chemical treatments that I was dispensing as a pharmacist. He invited me to come to a Parker Seminar in Dallas, Texas in March of 1992 so that I could meet more chiropractors and learn more about what they do. He was acquainted with Dr. Jim Parker and many of the other Parker disciples of that time and I got to meet Dr. Jim and sit in on a few of the classes. I also visited the campus at Parker College. Needless to say, I was impressed.

In May of 1992 Angi and I got married. In August of 1992 we quit our jobs and moved to Dallas, Texas, where I began to attend a Parker College of Chiropractic. I graduated from there in September of 1995 Summa Cum Laude and have been practicing chiropractic ever since. I have a home office in a rural suburb near Pittsburgh and have thoroughly enjoyed helping the thousands of patients that have come to me over these past almost 20 years. They say that when you love what you do work is not work and that is exactly how I feel about chiropractic. I still do the continuing education and maintain my pharmacy licenses in Pennsylvania and West Virginia. This knowledge allows me to stay informed with the ever-increasing number of medications that many of my patients are on. It has also allowed me to suggest changes to them and their medical doctors when the need for these medications was no longer necessary. I have a great respect for my colleagues in the medical and pharmaceutical professions. I feel that most of them are there for all the right reasons and that is to do the right thing for the patient. It is the business of health care that has gone the wrong way. But that is a subject for another time. My hope is that there will be more and more collaboration between chiropractors and those that practice orthodox medicine. Together we can do great things for the patients that need us which would greatly enhance their quality of life and also reduce total health care costs. These collaborations are occurring and my hope is that they will continue and accelerate. In the meantime I go to work every day with love and service to help my patients feel the power of their innate intelligence.

Chippewa Chiropractic Clinic

2401 Darlington Rd.

Beaver Falls, PA 15010

Phone: (724) 843-7255

Fax: (724) 843-2254

www.chippewachiropracticclinic.com

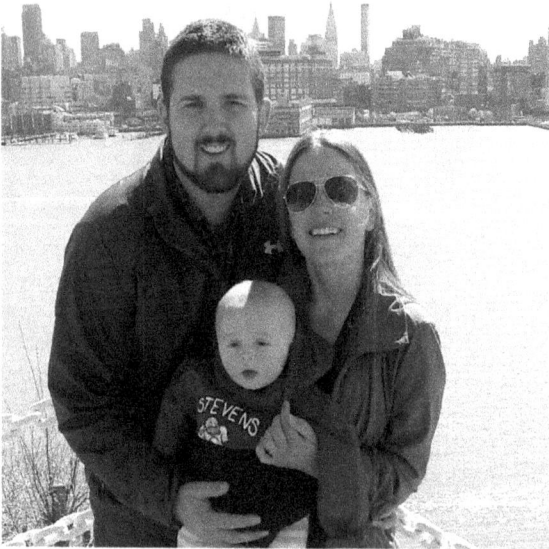

Dr. David Decker, D.C.

"Focusing on Lacrosse and Chiropractic"

Perhaps you think of baseball as America's sport, but lacrosse has been played in America for several hundred years. Native Americans would use crafted wooden sticks with a leather net to carry a ball across large areas of land in a scoring competition. The Iroquois people described lacrosse as a gift to us from the Creator, to be played for his enjoyment and as a medicine game for healing the people. As the game of lacrosse grew in America in the late 19th century, it became a regulated field game played between universities from Maryland to New York. The development of lacrosse equipment and the crafted stick - especially in the last 25 years - has enabled the small rubber ball to reach speeds up to 100mph with incredible accuracy. With this said, the skills of the lacrosse goalkeeper have had to be raised to a new level. Armed with a slightly wider stick and a few extra pads, the goalkeeper is often credited with perhaps having a few screws loose in order to take the position. And they're probably right, but I couldn't afford to play hockey growing up, and lacrosse was finally my chance to make amazing saves like my favorite hockey goalies of the time. Little did I know that I would succeed to become a collegiate goalkeeper.

In order to protect the 6ft x 6ft lacrosse goal, you need to have your eye on the ball and stop shots that other players instinctively jump out of the way for. But, to be great it's not as simple as removing the distractions. You can't simply make distractions go away so that all you see is the ball. It's all about focus. The player's gaze must be so focused that the distractions simply don't exist because the target is all you can see. You have to cut away the extraneous information to truly see. Little did I know, I was already growing the mind of a Chiropractor.

I received a full ride scholarship to play Division 1 lacrosse for Hofstra University. The plan was to weight lift all Summer to develop my strength and head out to Long Island in September. I hurt my back squatting a few weeks before I was to leave. To make a long story short, I tried my best but the pain became too much and the weakness in my left leg was affecting my ability to play. For the first time in my life, I had to quit lacrosse. I decided to focus on academics and transferred to Stevens Institute of Technology. Sure they had a decent Division 3 lacrosse team, but I was doubting my ability to play again so it didn't seem like a reality to get back in the goal. All I wanted was to walk without pain.

I remember the first day that I became a chiropractor. But to understand that day, you need to understand the last few months. First, I had seen an orthopedist. He sat across the room during our one minute examination and without even touching me, told me I had a disc problem. Despite the MRI not demonstrating any disc problems, we decided I needed a discal injection at L5-S1. Of course it did not work. The physical therapists and athletic trainers did their best to make sure I was applying ice and stretching. Of course it did not work. I wanted an answer. I decided to go to another physical therapist. This was the first day that I became a chiropractor. I met the doctor and asked politely if she would do an exam on me first without learning from my intake paperwork what my chief symptom was. I did not want to tell her I had low back pain just to be given a reflex response that I had been given before by other practitioners. I wanted the doctor to find the dysfunction, because it seemed to me to make more sense that the underlying dysfunction should be corrected. What I know now is that what I wanted was Chiropractic. She refused to do that for obvious medicolegal reasons which I completely agree with and understand now. But it worked out well because the next place I went to was where I should have gone to first, my Chiropractor's office.

With chiropractic care, the dysfunction was corrected. I played for Stevens for three years and was an NCAA All American all three of those years. The women's team at Stevens also had a fantastic player who was a Biomedical Engineer Major and All-American star, and she was cute too. We both thought it would be a great idea to date. A few years later, we both thought it would be a great idea to go to Parker University to continue our education and become Doctors of Chiropractic. With a one year old in the picture now, my wife and I have a successful clinic in New Jersey.

Perhaps you think of modern medicine when it comes to American Healthcare, but Chiropractic is America's true Healthcare. It may not be a multibillion dollar industry, but Chiropractic is a Science, Philosophy, and Art grounded into this nation's soil by the caring, dedicated providers who make it the pride of American ingenuity and determinism. Chiropractic works and will continue to work because we have focus. When it comes to patients, we focus on loving service. When it comes to performing, we focus on the detection, analysis, and adjustment of Chiropractic Subluxation. Lacrosse taught me how to focus. Chiropractic will teach me how focus can change the world.

New Jersey Nerve Activation Center

18 Main St.

Robbinsville, NJ 08691

Phone: (609) 981-7560

Email: contact@NJnerve.com

www.njnerve.com

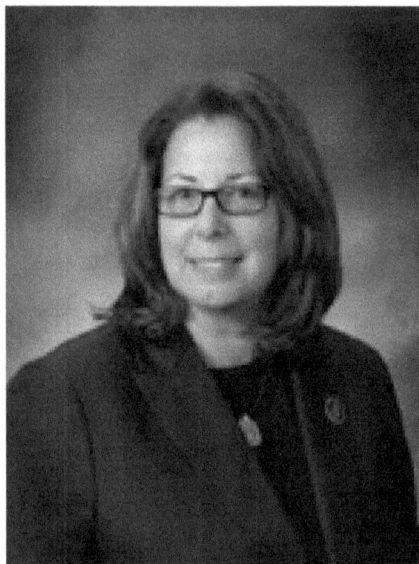

Jayne Moschella, D.C.

"How I Became a Chiropractor"

I was born in 1961 the youngest of 3 children to an Italian American family in a small town 8 miles from Manhattan called Lodi, NJ.

Caregiver:

I was a very good student, daughter, sister and friend. As a grade school child my mom and dad would sometimes keep me home from school to help care for my ailing grandmother. We were very close and I loved helping her get through sick and painful days. It was common for me to be the helper in most situations.

As I became a teenager my brother who was just 15 months older became addicted to drugs. I again stayed home from school to care for him, and later his baby (his teen girlfriend died in his arms when their baby was 6 months old). Care giving was second nature to me by this time.

Vocational pursuits:

My first love was art; painting, drawing, sculpting, photography, etc. I won several art awards through high school. I was given a scholarship to the School of Visual Arts in NYC, but quickly lost it due to missing too much school in my senior year of high school.

Once I graduated from high school, I began a series of interesting jobs: bartender, roadie for an all-girl rock band, factory worker, IT clerk, even fast food… One day in May 1984 (5 years after my high school graduation) I was invited to my cousin's college graduation at Penn State. She and I grew up like sisters and best friends but grew apart when she went off to college and I stayed behind to drift aimlessly. That weekend was quite the eye opener for me. The new college graduates were fun, excited, full of promise, and I was deflated and disgusted with my lack of focus.

Fate would intervene… while drinking too much with the grads, I was messing around and fell on my back and hurt my neck… I could hardly turn my head. My friend took me to his chiropractor, Dr. W., in Stanhope, NJ, and she was amazing. I was intrigued. She was not much older than me; she had her own practice and was so knowledgeable and caring. I asked her a million questions and she took me under her wing. That was May, by that September I was in college for pre-chiropractic studies (pre-med).

In spite of my cousins, who are medical doctors, asking me "Why don't you become a real doctor, you are so smart!" I stayed with it and in December 1989 I graduated from Palmer Chiropractic College in Davenport, Iowa.

So many amazing things happened through my 15 years in practice. I was fortunate to have practiced in California, North Carolina, Virginia, New Jersey, and Florida. I continue to hold 5 state licenses and hope to one day get back to practicing as a physician. While practicing in Deerfield Beach, FL, my path was changed when I happened upon the Florida College of Natural Health. I wandered into the school on a whim and was soon teaching anatomy and physiology too, soon to be, massage therapists and estheticians. This began my path to teaching the "wonders of chiropractic" to hundreds of students for more than 5 years. From teaching I was offered a position at a new college in Fort Lauderdale where I was asked to develop the first in the US accredited Bachelor of Science Degree in Alternative Medicine. The program became the fastest growing and largest program at the university. Through this program we get to teach a college course called "Introduction to Chiropractic" as well as many other courses designed to teach different approaches to the mind-body-spirit connection. As the Vice President of Academic Affairs for Everglades University, I oversaw more than 1,600 graduates and over 800 were from the Alternative Medicine program. I have the great fortune to be able to extol the great profession and philosophies of chiropractic. Many graduates of the alternative medicine program have gone on to chiropractic school.

I have seen so many positive changes in the American thirst for "heath" care as opposed to "sick" care, preventative treatments, Complementary and Alternative Medicine, naturopathy, homeopathy, acupuncture and nutrition. One of the most profound experiences in my professional career as a practicing physician was working with my sister and her infertility. She had been trying all different therapies, drugs, and treatments for 4 years to no avail. I asked her to go off all medications and treatments and I started adjusting her regularly. She became pregnant 2 months later! I have treated patients with everything from musculoskeletal issues to mood and emotional disorders with positive results. So many fellow chiropractors have inspired me to continue educating everyone I come in contact with about this amazing profession. I had the great honor to learn from Dr. Burl Pettibon at his home in Washington State as well as in the California office where I was an associate way back in the late 80's early 90's. What an inspiration!

I find myself now as the Vice President of Academic Affairs for Everglades University where I integrate chiropractic principles with cutting-edge new academic programs such as Alternative and Renewable Energy Management, Crisis and Disaster Management, green building courses, Land and energy Management, and Public Health Administration with a Concentration in Complementary and Alternative Medicine. These exciting programs fit perfectly with the new world order for a cleaner environment and health care preventive options.

I also am extremely proud to serve on the Board of Trustees for Parker University in Texas.

Dr. Jayne Moschella

Email: jaynemoschella@gmail.com

Phone: (954) 729-1100

**SMITH
CHIROPRACTIC**

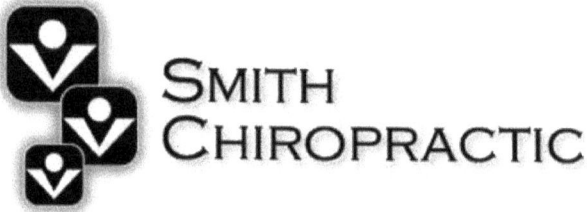

Dr. Oliver "Bud" Smith, D.C.

"My Father..."

My father, Dr Oliver R. Smith Sr. graduated from Texas Chiropractic College in 1938. He opened his practice shortly after, I believe on the third floor of the Abdou Bldg in downtown El Paso, just before he enlisted in the Army Air Corp where he flew C-46's and 47's over Okinawa in WWII. Considering the public opinion of Chiropractic at that time, he knew opening a practice would be an uphill battle. He chose to be downtown because at the time, it had the greatest concentration of people in El Paso. His office hours were Monday- Friday from 7am-6pm and Saturday from 8am-12 noon. For roughly six months he had no patients... not one. Despite that, he came to the office everyday dressed in his suit, on time, and waited. At the end of each day he never closed his door early despite not having a patient this entire time. One day Dad was in the hallway in front of his office and noticed a janitor cleaning the floors. Dad said something to him but the man did not respond. My Dad having been raised on a ranch was also fluent in Spanish and thinking the gentleman did not speak English spoke to him again in Spanish. Again the man did not respond. Shortly after, the man turned and saw my Dad standing there. The janitor spoke to Dad and in the course of their conversation told him he had gradually lost his hearing after a car accident years earlier and had learned to read lips. Dad, thinking about Dr. DD Palmer and the Harvey Lillard story, told the man while he himself had never treated someone with hearing loss, he was aware that Chiropractic adjustments had help similar conditions in the past. The man said he greatly appreciated the offer but being a janitor he had no means to pay Dad for his services. As an interesting note, in 1938 Dad was charging one dollar for an adjustment. Dad said he understood but wanted to try to help the man anyway. So Dad started treating the man and after 6 or so weeks of treatment, the janitor's hearing gradually returned. Dad remembers it was a Saturday and he had just finished treating the man. The gentleman, as he did after every treatment, expressed his appreciation for what Dad had done for him. Again he apologized for not being able to pay my Dad anything, but promised he was going to make sure he told everyone he knew and everyone who would listen, about what Chiropractic and Dad had done for him. Monday morning Dad arrived at his office at the usual time. When the elevator doors opened he was surprised to see a long line of people standing in the hallway. Dad thought maybe a new business had opened but as he rounded the corner to his office he noticed that they were all standing in line waiting at his front door. Dad opened his door and remembers never sitting down the whole day with an office filled with patients. Dad continued to practice for 56 years. I joined him in 1975 and I never remember him having a slow day the rest of his career.

Smith Chiropractic LLC.

1417 N Brown St

El Paso, TX 79902

Phone: (915) 533-2225

Fax: (915) 533-0974

Email: drsmithsoffice@sbcglobal.net

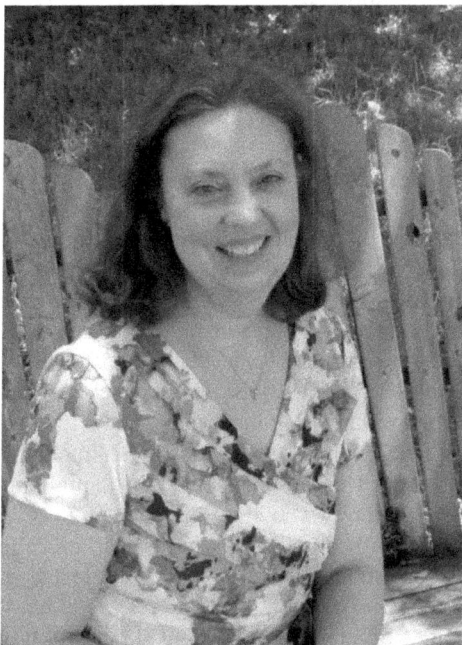

Dr. Mary White, D.C.

"I am Proud to Say…"

I am proud to say that I come from a chiropractic family that lived some interesting pieces of chiropractic history. My father's great uncle was a forward-thinking chiropractor and passionate proponent of the chiropractic profession. Dr. Godfrey Frutiger taught at the first chiropractic college, Palmer School of Chiropractic, in Davenport, Iowa, for 13 years in the early part of the last century. He taught alongside B.J. Palmer, who is considered the Developer of the profession. (B.J. Palmer's father, D. Daniel Palmer, founded the chiropractic profession in 1895.) The story goes that whenever Uncle Godfrey visited, you could expect to hear preaching on the philosophy of chiropractic!

As my father grew up, his Uncle Godfrey treated him for migraines, low back pain, and scoliosis. But, that was not my father's first exposure to the world of chiropractic. When my father was almost 2 years old, he contracted polio during one of the epidemics that hit southern Minnesota in the late 1920's. He exhibited paralysis from the waist down, which included severe digestive disturbances. My grandparents sought the help of a local chiropractor, Dr. Chapman, who worked with him until the condition resolved. This was considered the family miracle. Most others in the community who had contracted polio at the time ended up permanently paralyzed. What was different about my father's experience compared to most others? He had chiropractic care. No one fully understood the "how's" at the time --- only that freeing the spine of interference, which allowed for proper nerve flow, brought healing and optimal function. Now, we know that an adjustment also has a positive impact on the immune system, which was likely a key factor in my father's full recovery.

Although the family background was mostly farming, it is no surprise that my father considered chiropractics as a career. Despite many hardships, he was able to begin his chiropractic education in 1946 at Northwestern Chiropractic College in St. Paul, MN. He graduated in a class of 12 in 1950 and had a successful practice for 43 years in Rochester, MN. The location for his practice made sense. Rochester was 15 miles from Pine Island, MN, where both my parents were born. However, this practice location was also destined to play a unique role in chiropractic history.

My father started his practice in a remodeled rooming house that was between the renowned Mayo Clinic, and the clinic's main hospital, St. Mary's Hospital. Our family lived in the upper stories of the house, and Dad converted the street-level basement to his office. If you went from St. Mary's to the Mayo Clinic, you went right by Dr. Raymond Brown, D.C.'s office. He tells the story that the original Mayo brothers, Will and Charlie, had a family member with a significant spinal dysfunction. When medical efforts could not help, they sought a chiropractor who was able to improve the condition. For that reason, Dad says that the Mayo's were always friendly to chiropractors, to the degree that my family received complete professional courtesy care at both the clinic and hospital up through my own birth in 1956.

In the late 1950's the atmosphere of professional support from medical doctors to chiropractors began to decline. The American Medical Association was becoming concerned that the growth of the chiropractic profession was a competitive threat. In the early 1960's the A.M.A. began a campaign to "contain and eliminate" chiropractors. In 1963, a Committee on Quackery adopted an ethical guideline that threatened members with loss of hospital privileges for any kind of professional interaction with a chiropractor. The propaganda and politics against chiropractors became nasty. The situation was so intense that several Mayo medical doctors, who were patients of my father, had to ask to come to his office at night, disguised, so as not to be recognized.

There were many difficult years as the chiropractic profession was continually attacked by the A.M.A. In 1976, a lawsuit alleging violation of anti-trust laws was filed against the A.M.A. It's conclusion in 1983 and re-trial in 1992 brought attention to the issue. The A.M.A. was forced to change its Code of Ethics to allow for professional exchange with chiropractors. However, in the years of propaganda against chiropractors, the reputation of the chiropractic profession suffered significant damage. Unfortunately, misinformation that was propagated decades ago endures today, and chiropractors still find themselves defending their profession. Overall acceptance has certainly improved since the "dark days", as my father calls them. Alternative healthcare is becoming more mainstream, and multi-disciplinary clinics with M.D.'s and D.C. working together are becoming more common. However, the lines of communication between medical doctors and chiropractors are still not as strong as they should be, and, unfortunately, it is the patient that suffers. Few are aware that the root of the problem goes back to old political issues.

Overall, during a time of turbulent professional politics, my father remained a very respected doctor even in the midst of the powerful Mayo Clinic medical world. Other chiropractors were fighting a very vocal war on the unfair treatment of the chiropractic profession. However, my father never participated in a battle. All he did was continue to treat patients with utmost integrity and devotion to their well-being. His quiet humility, professionalism, and successful treatments gave him a powerful reputation. In spite of the A.M.A.'s threats to its members, the orthopedic and neurological departments of the Mayo Clinic continued to share information and patients with my father. One of the Mayo doctors admitted at a gathering that my father, Dr. Brown, was their "go-to" doctor if all else failed.

Most chiropractors don't know my father's name or much about him. There is nothing flashy about my dad. But, he was one of the quiet heroes who modeled the best of the chiropractic profession at a strategic place and time in history. He didn't even know what impact he was making by being who he was and where he was. His hard work and devotion to his solo practice made such a difference to so many and in so many ways. I have always been so proud of him.

Fast forward.

It was the first day of school. I was a high school biology teacher, and I had asked my sophomore students to write out their goals. What would you like to be doing in 3 years, 5 years, or 10 years? I walked around the room, reading the student's responses. I got to the desk of a girl, Nicole, who I knew was the daughter of a local chiropractor because of her recognizable last name. I looked at what she had written, and I felt chills.

You see, Nicole had written that she wanted to be a chiropractor. My first thought was that I was happy for her. She already knew what she wanted, and she would be carrying out a family tradition. My second thought was one of revelation. I realized in that moment that I, too, wanted to be a chiropractor! Chiropractics was also my family tradition. I knew in my heart that I had always wanted to follow in my father's footsteps, but life had gotten in the way.

My third thought was that of sadness. Now, I knew what I wanted, but it seemed impossible. I was 38 years old, my income was a necessity, and my husband's job was established in Austin, TX. The nearest chiropractic college was 200 miles away. Become a chiropractor at this point in life? How could that ever happen? But my dream was so strong. I just started to pray for a miracle.

As I continued to teach over the next three years, slowly but surely, doors and windows began to open. I found out that there were government loans that would completely cover the significant cost of a health professional degree. I also learned that, with my degrees and background in science, my acceptance at a chiropractic college was guaranteed. As the impossible started to hint of possibility, I dared to think about the logistics of going back to school. In an act of generosity, my father-in-law agreed to let me live in his 1940-era rent house in Dallas in return for making it livable again. A plan emerged where I would go to Parker College of Chiropractic in Dallas, live in the Dallas house during the week, and commute back to my Austin home on the weekends.

In the spring of 1997, I received my acceptance letter for Parker College of Chiropractic, and I turned in my resignation for my teaching job. I started classes at the community college to refresh my memory and get back in the habit of being a student. I moved to Dallas over the Christmas break, and in January, 1998, I was ready to start my chiropractic career. -- Or, so I thought!

As I began my 45 minute drive through Dallas to my first day of classes, I was shaking like a leaf. During that commute, the impossibility of this major career change started to take over in my mind. I thought, "What am doing? Am I crazy? I gave up a good job. I'm 41 years old, and twenty years older than all the other students. What was I thinking?!" As I drove closer to the school, I became physically ill as nerves took over.

When I arrived at my building, I could hardly walk up the steps to my classroom. Ahead of me loomed big double doors. With effort, I slowly pushed the door open and dared to look inside. What awaited me was unbelievable. My eyes locked on the first face I saw. It was Nicole!

What a profound moment! I knew at once that I was in the right place. My prayers for a miracle over three years had been answered beyond my dreams. And, the miracle continued. Nicole and I graduated together. Amazingly, even with the burden of having commuted over 77,000 miles during the course of my chiropractic education, I was still able to come in second in my class. As Salutatorian, I was asked to give a speech at graduation and share my miraculous journey of faith with over 500 attendees. It also gave me a platform to honor my father, who had been such a quiet, but strong advocate for the chiropractic profession for so many years.

Now, 15 years later, I still get chills when I think of the day I read Nicole's paper. I have loved every minute of being a chiropractor and building my practice. When my patients refer to me as their friend and healer, I am humbled. I also delight in the fact that my father, who is 88, now lives near me and is able to see the dream that he started in me come to fruition. In my practice, I continue to witness miracles, both small and large, every day. It is a true blessing to be a chiropractor!

Chiropractic Clinic

206A Laurel Drive

Round Rock, TX 78664

Phone: (512) 248-8700

www.RoundRockChiroHeaven.com

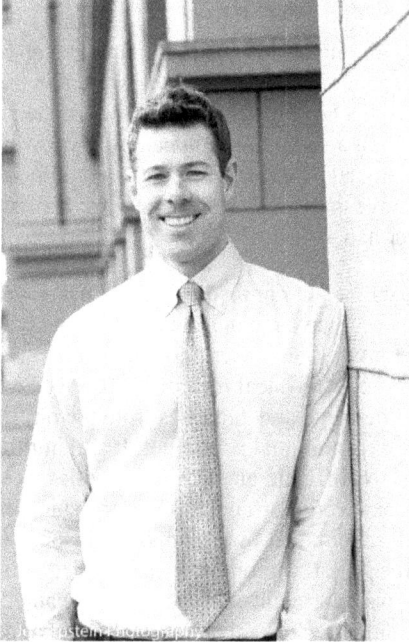

Dr. Adam Jacobs

D.C., C.C.S.P., A.R.T.

"... We were Meant to Move..."

My name is Dr. Adam Jacobs, and my chiropractic story began at the age of 17 when I suffered a herniated disc in my low back from a wakeboarding injury. For those who don't know what wakeboarding is, it is a surface water sport where an individual on a wakeboard, which is like a snowboard, is towed behind a boat going between 15-35 MPH. The objective of this sport is for the rider to get big air and perform tricks jumping over wake to wake. I had been wakeboarding for over 5 years and had taken many bad falls, but it was this last big fall I took that herniated my disc. Immediately, I felt a sharp, burning pain in my low back that traveled down my right leg. My muscles went into spasm, and I could barely move and get back into the boat. It was the worse pain that I have ever had.

After my injury I sought out medical care. First, I went to my primary doctor who gave me muscle relaxers and pain killers. However, after a week on prescription medication and not getting any better, I visited a physical therapist. I received ice, heat, e-stimulation, ultrasound, and exercises from the physical therapist, but the results were minimal pain relief. It still hurt to walk, sitting and sleeping were difficult, and simple activities like putting on my pants or socks were a struggle. It was the summer time after I graduated high school, and I was supposed to start my college basketball career in a few months. I was worried and frustrated. Growing up, I was a straight-A student, and I wanted to become a sports doctor, either a physical therapist or an orthopedist. I had tried physical therapy but had yet to see an orthopedist. The next step for me was to go to an orthopedist, since the previous treatments did not work out. At the orthopedist, I received an epidural into my low back but found minimal relief; in fact, I felt worse afterwards for a few days. The orthopedist said that if the epidural didn't work, then surgery would be the next step. Summer was nearing its end and fall basketball was about to commence. At the time, I thought there was no chance I was going to be able to play. I could barely walk without having pain in my low back; how was I supposed to play basketball? I was scared and frustrated and didn't know what to do next. My only option was to either get surgery or try chiropractic.

Boy, was I glad I decided to try chiropractic! Going into the visit, I was scared to have my back adjusted; was it going to hurt or break a bone? What I got was a smooth, non-painful adjustment by a skilled doctor. I found relief immediately following my first adjustment. It was short lived, but it was hope. I continued to get adjusted and continued the exercises that the chiropractor and previous physical therapist gave me. By the end of summer when it was time to start college, I was able to run, jump, and play basketball again. I had avoided that path toward surgery and decided at that point that I wanted to attend chiropractic school after my undergraduate studies. It was the best decision I have ever made.

Now, 16 years later, I have multiple chiropractic clinics in the San Francisco Bay Area and have been voted top chiropractor in the Bay Area by both Yelp and ABC 7 News Best of the Bay. I now get to help patients just like I was who had tried other forms of treatment without seeing success and who have been told they needed surgery. I am still able to play basketball and wakeboard, though not as good as I once was in my college days, but I am still able to do what I love.

As a chiropractor, I know that the key to keeping your back and body healthy is keeping it flexible and stable - that means being strong and mobile. We were meant to move not sit; we were meant to stand tall not slouch. If you move correctly and your spine and joints move correctly, then there is not going to be stress and dysfunction, which mean you stay healthy. This is something I teach my patients, and I incorporate stretches and exercises along with regular spinal adjustments and muscle work to the body in order for it to reach its optimal health. By doing so, I am enabling my patients to take control of their back and musculoskeletal problems, which help them to achieve and maintain the healthy lifestyle they have always aimed for.

SF Custom Chiropractic

425 Washington St, STE 100

San Francisco, CA 94111

Phone: 415-788-8700

www.sfcustomchiro.com

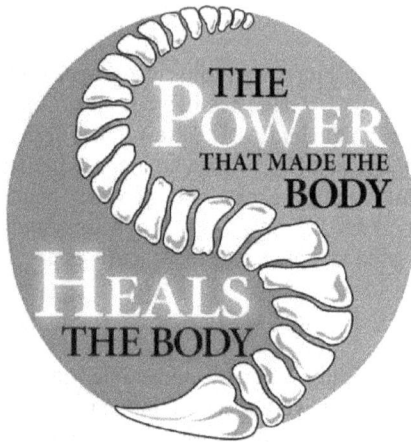

Dr. Bobbie Stowe, D.C.

"My Story to Discovery"

I was born in 1953 with several genetic flaws; probably due to the fact that both of my parents smoked unfiltered Camel cigarettes like they were chimneys. Not only was I exposed during pregnancy, but continued to have to breathe second-hand smoke until I left my parent's home at the age of 18. But my parents didn't know any better; it was just what people did back then. As a matter of fact, TV News Broadcasters and even medical doctors did ads for TV and print, showing how great it was to smoke this or that brand of cigarette. My, how times have changed and with it, our understanding of health. We still don't know all we need to know about the body or else, we wouldn't be dealing with so many chronic diseases. And make no mistake about it; chronic diseases represent the vast majority of our medical costs today and are expected to continue to rise, at an alarming rate, for the foreseeable future. But if I could improve just one thing, it would be the communication and understanding between the medical and CAM providers. There is absolutely a need for both professionals and this is my story of how and why I became a Chiropractor.

So at 3 days old, I had a spinal tumor removed from my tail bone. The doctor told my parents there was a 50% chance that I would never walk, but he was proven wrong. Then shortly after the surgery, I started having extremely severe pain that would cause me to scream and cry in such pain that my parents couldn't even take me out in public. This pain would occur 2-4 times a year; it would come without warning and it would leave without warning. Medical doctors were completely stumped and couldn't find anything wrong with me, but the pain continued until one day, I started urinating blood and an old family doctor finally told my parents there was something wrong with my kidneys and after seeing a urologist and finally having surgery, I was fixed. I had lived with that pain for 13 years. Then again, shortly after that, I started experiencing extreme low back pain that would leave me in bed for days at a time. Multiple visits to many medical doctors, an untold number of tests and nothing was found, until I met my first chiropractor; I was 35 years old. He diagnosed me with a "congenital broken back", a spondylolisthesis and after two visits and a couple of adjustments, my pain was gone, and it has never returned. Thus started my experience with chiropractic and my eventual career change to become a Doctor of Chiropractic. Unfortunately, my story, while different in specifics, still remains the model and approach in our healthcare industry today. And it is truly a sad state of affairs when all the medical community has to offer are drugs and surgery. Doesn't it seem that there should be more to offer patients? How about a true understanding of what is causing the patient's pain or disease? Has any medical doctor ever said to a patient, "let's see if we can find out WHY, you are presenting with your symptoms?" I think not.

I left a fairly lucrative job in the financial industry because of my dissatisfaction and lack of fulfillment in what I was doing. I had actually been pre-med in the 70's but even back then, became disenchanted with the direction that medicine was heading. So after leaving the business field, my wife and I agreed that my joy and love of helping people might best be suited in the medical field, but not as an MD, but rather a DC. So at 49 years old, I started my journey at Texas Chiropractic College in Pasadena TX, just outside of Houston, my home town.

During my education, besides learning to understand the body and how it REALLY functions, I was taught the art and science of the adjustment and how adjustments really help the body to heal. You see, the body wants to be healthy, but too many times, internal and external forces push the body in directions that are harmful. Stress, inflammation, injury, and drugs are unfortunately becoming all too common place in today's society, causing demands and extracting punishment that the body, simply can't deal with. Doctors of Chiropractic understand this and almost every one of us, focus on helping our patients not by just the adjustments we provide, but also by the recommendations, testing and counselling we do, in our effort to help our patients understand the importance of how to live a more healthy life.

While at TCC, I also started learning about Functional Medicine. This is a branch of what is called CAM – complementary and alternative medicine – of which chiropractic is also a part. FM utilizes special, objective laboratory testing in order to determine what the functional cause of disease might be. What I look for is cellular dysfunction; in other words, what has happened at the cellular level, that has caused a change in the body, that has caused symptoms or diseases in the body. This is an entirely different approach than allopathic or "modern" medicine. Visit a medical doctor with symptoms and most times, you leave with a prescription or two, but NEVER with the understanding of why or what actually caused your symptoms or disease; just a drug. And it is not entirely their fault. In medical school, they simply are not taught to find the cause of a symptom or disease. And there are two other issues. First, they don't have enough time to spend with a patient to uncover what might be the cause of a condition and the second, is money. I know it sounds disturbing, but medicine is a business and medical doctors, like everyone else, need to make a living. Today, in 2015, it is extremely expensive to staff and run a medical office. I realize they are dealing with a life, but at the end of the day, medical doctors have two things and only two things to offer; drugs or surgery. That is simply all they have. But doesn't the patient have a right to know what might be causing their condition, especially if there are alternatives to drugs and surgery?

Something I ask all my FM patients is, were you born with a genetic defect or were you hit by a mac truck? If the answer is no, then something in your body changed and my job, my passion, is to try and find out what and why. Many times, using laboratory testing, if I can find out what and or why, cellular change has occurred, then there are many natural protocols that can help the body to restore its nature balance and health. For example, I have many patients who come in with fatigue, brain fog, lack of mood or intimacy, and can't sleep well. Almost everyone has seen a medical doctor and almost every one of them was diagnosed with some form of anxiety or mild depression and given an anti-depressive medication. But the thing is, that these people aren't depressed and they know it; they can feel it, there is something wrong, something has changed, but they, the patient, don't know what to do, and neither do the medical doctors. But I do. I have a very specific, objective laboratory test that will show a problem with their adrenal glands and once a protocol is started, EVERYONE of those patients start getting better. The secret is that I listened to the patient and knew what test to run and then how to provide the body with what it needed to regain balance.

As I stated before, the body wants to be healthy and in balance and the best example I can give someone is to understand how the body would heal a broken bone. When someone breaks a bone, the body – all by itself – immediately starts the healing process. It doesn't need a doctor or nurse or anyone, it simply knows to start that healing on its own. Now, a medical professional might set the bone so it will heal straight, but even if that bone needs surgery, the body is what heals the bone. But that is not the most remarkable part of the story. The most remarkable part of this story is that the body knew when to STOP HEALING. Please re-read that sentence. The body not only knew when to start the healing but it also knew when to stop the healing. The body wants to be in balance and health!

My entire professional life is now dedicated to helping my patients to understand that they can become healthy. Medical doctors are the most important and necessary professionals on the planet, in an acute medial situation; but at the same time, they are the most ill-equipped professionals, once that acute condition becomes chronic. That is where chiropractors and other CAM providers are at their best. We listen to our patients and understand the underlying workings of the body and our profession is trained to handle many chronic conditions; not just pain.

And just like your professional DC, doctors who practice Functional Medicine are simply taking the CAM approach to a different level. People who have never experienced an adjustment are amazed at how wonderful and relaxed they feel after that first visit to a chiropractor. And the same holds true for my FM patients. They tell me that they never thought they could feel this good again and many of them are able to stop taking those drugs that they were told, they would be on forever.

Chiropractic has changed my life and given me the freedom and love of getting out of bed every morning, knowing that today, I just might help someone else, become healthy.

Dr. Bobbie Stowe, DC

2400 Augusta Dr. Suite 210

Houston, TX 77057

Phone: 713-667-6656

www.westuchiropractic.com

www.functionalmedicineofhouston.com

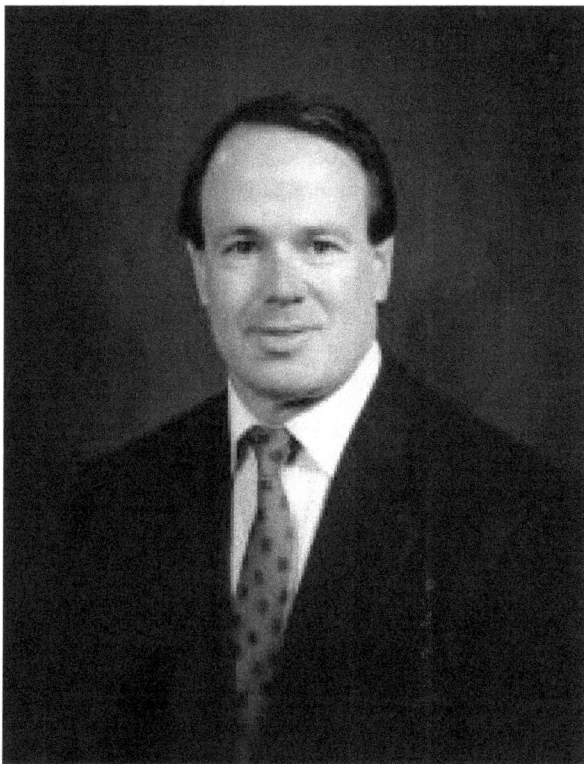

Dr. Jack Dolbin

"...The Best Things in Life Are Not Things..."

A few years ago, I was standing in the long line at the funeral home to offer my condolences to the family of my friend Dr. Douglas N. Howe. Doug was a fellow Chiropractor and the last of a generation of Chiropractors that included my grandfather and father. He was 83. As I stood in line I was reminded of that day in December 1968 when I stood on the receiving end of the same line of those offering their sympathies. I was 19 and my dad had just died, he was 49. My dad was a Chiropractor. In the line of well wishers were two state senators, one United States congressman, the mayor of Pottsville, Pa. and many that society would label as important people. But the people that most impressed me and have left an indelible impression in my mind of that day, now 42 years ago, were those who came in bib overalls, the farmers with dirt under their fingernails, the miners who just came out of the pits with coal dirt imbedded in their faces and tears streaking their hardened faces. These were two fisted drinkers and fighters, tough men in a tough world, weeping. These were my dad's patients. They came to show their respect and express their grief. My dad died in his office treating a patient. The medical examiner diagnosed his death as a result of a dissecting abdominal aneurism, I diagnosed it as exhaustion. There were many who came up to me, his oldest son, that evening to express their condolences but the one I remember most was the elderly lady who hugged me very close, not wanting to let go and said repeatedly," What are we to do now". My dad literally gave his life for his patients and they all knew it.

My dad practiced in a town bordering the coal region and farming region of Pennsylvania. When I was a young boy he would take me to work with him on weekends. I had an ulterior motive. Mrs. Kimmel had an ice cream shop on the first floor below my dad's office. She always had a cone waiting for me. My dad's routine was to treat patients during his office hours, then get dinner at a local diner before making his house calls to the local farms. I recall the day I decided to become a Chiropractor, I was 6. It was snowing and my dad pulled up to this particular farm. He had to park out on the street and as we walked through the snow covered field, he carried me on his shoulders. He treated the entire family and we then walked back to our 49 Chrysler. When we got in the car I mentioned that he did not get paid. He simply reminded me that all they had for dinner that night was a pot of potatoes. I complained that he should have been paid something. Stopping the car on that snowy road he put his hand on my shoulder and said "When I get to heaven I will get everything that is coming to me." When we got home I told my mom that I had that day decided to become a Chiropractor.

In 1984, after graduating from National College and retiring from a 6 year career in the NFL with the Denver Broncos which included starting 67 consecutive games including Super Bowl 12, I decided to move my family back to my home in central Pennsylvania. I opened up a modest office and began serving those patients who sought my services. My grandfather opened a similar office in 1921 and my dad in 1947. What I found was most encouraging. I did not have to defend Chiropractic. Since 1921 this small coal region town had been served by a continuum of great Chiropractors, I was just an extension of doctors like my grandfather, dad, Doug Howe, and Harry Hoffman. Doctors who treated patients, not benefits, and left a long legacy of quality care and paved the way for the future generations of Chiropractors. Doctors like my daughter who graduated from National in 2007. These young Chiropractors will practice in my shadow as I have now for 38 years, practiced in my dad's. My dad never got an award. There was no plaque on his office wall, only his diploma and discharge papers for his military service. He was never recognized as " Chiropractor of the Year", the award the various state association leaders give to each other at state conventions. But, he left the profession a bit better than he found it and left a legacy of grateful patients.

So as I hugged Dr. Doug Howes daughter a few weeks ago, I offered my sympathies but also my thanks. Thanks for her dad for representing the profession with grace and dignity and leaving it a bit better than he found it and paving the way for my generation to continue in his wake.

As General Douglas MacArthur said in his famous West Point speech "the shadows are lengthening for me now". Someday I too will pass over Jordan. I would hope in the context of my professional life as a Chiropractor I would have left the profession a bit better and maybe some elderly lady will say at my funeral "what are we to do now".

In 38 years of practice I have learned the truth of the statement, "The best things in life are not things".

Schuylkill Medical Center

700 Schuylkill Manor Rd.

Pottsville, PA 17901

www.proseriesseminars.com

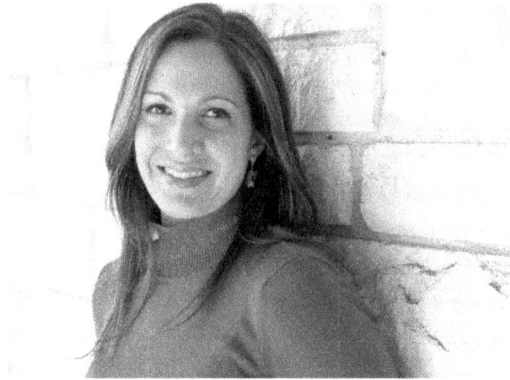

Dr. Julia Pinkerton, D.C.

"My Chiropractic Story Begins…"

My chiropractic story begins with my mother. Mom was about six months pregnant with me when she started having some of the aches and pains that can be associated with pregnancy. Some of her new friends in our rural community recommended that she see a chiropractor. I was lucky that my mother was Brazilian and had none of the stigma associated with going to a chiropractor because she had never heard of it before, so she made an appointment with the closest one she could find.

While she was there the chiropractor taught her the importance of the spine and nervous system, which controls every process in the body. It would be coming in to play during the birth process and he assured her that the birth would be better if she continued to get adjusted as it can reduce labor time, painful labor and it is easier on the baby. He also told her that the birth process can be a traumatic not only to her, but to her baby, and that she should get her baby checked as soon as possible after the birth too.

A few months later I was born and it was quite traumatic for both mom and I. She had back labor, so I had my skull banging on her sacrum for a long period of time. They even had to use forceps a bit as well (the jerks). So at ten days old she took me in to get checked for the first time and I received my first chiropractic adjustment.

My second adjustment came after a nasty fall down our wooden basement stairs in my walker. And that's how it was growing up. When something happened, mom took me to my chiropractor or my Naturopath, who also did an occasional manipulation of the spine. They were my two primary care physicians. I was never seriously ill, never went to the hospital, and barely ever saw a medical doctor.

In 1999 mom got the opportunity to open a branch of her sales company in Brazil. The idea was for me to stay a year, meet my family, learn the language and then come back for undergrad. My grandmother had 10 siblings so we had about 30 cousins our age waiting with arms open. Brazilians men are warm, beautiful and charming and I fell in love with it all. After living there for eight months I went to my mother crying saying, "I don't want to go back!" They were of course more than happy to have me stay and so it was decided. Now the question was, "What do I do with my life?"

Through my mom's networking activities with the Rotary Club she met a chiropractor that came to speak in her group, the first she had met in Brazil. He told her about the first chiropractic program in Brazil starting at Centro Universitario Feevale, only 45 minutes away. We were all so excited to go get adjusted! As we were there the professor looked at me and asked if I had considered being a chiropractor.

The thought was amazing! No, I hadn't thought of it. I had grown up under chiropractic care, I loved biology and science and hated blood. It was perfect for me! Mom was very encouraging as well (mostly because she just wanted a chiropractor in the family I'm pretty sure).

Now in Brazil the school system is different. You graduate high school at 17 and you have to choose which profession it is that you want to study at that time. There is a big test called the Vestibular that is over everything they learn in high school, which was: Portuguese, Portuguese literature, Portuguese history, writing (in Portuguese), calculus, biology, physics, chemistry and English (Yes! One I was sure I could ace). Needless to say, I was freaked out!

But hard work and perseverance pay off (well, that, and a six month crash course on all those subjects) and guess what? I passed on the first try! Then I was set, ready to start my chiropractic adventure! In Brazil it's a 5-year bachelor degree+ program, with chiropractic school and undergrad rolled together. I had an amazing philosophy teacher my first year in school (Dr. Marcos Palmeira who currently practices in Salvador, Brazil). He taught us about Innate Intelligence, how the power that made the body could heal the body and that vertebral subluxations can interfere in this amazing healing potential. I then read Chiropractic Philosophy by Joseph B. Strauss and I was hooked! This was what I was meant to do! I finally had a calling!

I also got to work with an amazing American couple there to teach and run the clinic by the name of Richard and Virginia Irby. I was one of their translators in the clinic so daily I got to translate chiropractic education to people that had never heard of anything of the sort. But it resonated with them and people started to travel from far and wide to come see these amazing American doctors that were really shaking things up and helping people heal like they had never seen before.

There I was cruising along through chiropractic school with not a care in the world, having the time of my life. The licensing agency of chiropractic education in the US came to give us a pilot exam to see how our education was going. It was then that I got to talk to one of the higher ups and ask him how I would go about getting licensed in the US once I was done with school. He looked at me with big eyes and paused before he said to me "You cannot get licensed in the US with the education you had here, unfortunately. The school here is not CCE (Council of Chiropractic Education) accredited."

I was in shock! It had never even crossed my mind that I may not be able to get licensed in my home country with the education I had just received. I obviously didn't do my due diligence in researching it, but accreditation and board licensing were not even part of my vocabulary when I began chiropractic school. I hadn't the foggiest idea of what any of it meant. But at that moment it meant that I could never practice in the States and I was crushed. Even though I loved Brazil, the thought of never being able to practice the profession that I loved in my own home country was too much for me to handle. With only six months left and only having clinic and my thesis to finish I completed the program with a cloud over my head.

I was determined to find a loophole. I knew there must be a way to get around it. I came back to the States on a mission. I contacted many of the presidents of chiropractic schools along with anyone else I could think of. I paid special attention to the president at the time of Palmer College of Chiropractic since it was through them that the course in Brazil had started and was affiliated with. I contacted the NBCE (National Board of Chiropractic Education), all to no avail. All everyone had to tell me was: you need to do chiropractic school again and not only that you need pre-requisites to get into our programs.

So I was faced with the decision. Should I do it all again, or do I chose something else? And I'm not going to lie, I faltered and almost chose to pursue another path. I was working in a very big and busy chiropractic practice in Vancouver, WA and getting my pre-requisites done at some of the local community colleges in my off times. I was working hard and studying and just got a little burned out. I thought, "If I'm really supposed to do this, would there be this many obstacles in my way? Maybe it just wasn't meant to be."

Luckily I was networking at the time and came across a life coach. "There is something I think I could enjoy doing," I thought to myself. I decided to hire her to see what it was all about and if I thought maybe it was a better endeavor than spending $150,000 (without the interest) and 4 years of my life on chiropractic school again. I was already 28 at the time, which would put me starting my career at the age of 32. The plan backfired though. Instead she actually helped me gain a better understanding of who I was, what I wanted to do and why I actually should pursue this career that I had come to love. And I was back on track again!

If you are someone who understands the chiropractic philosophy, you know how important it is in practicing a vitalistic chiropractic practice, which is what I always wanted and why I really fell in love with the profession. This philosophy looks not at what is wrong with the body, like a pain or symptom, but what is right in the body. The truth is that our body's all have the capacity to heal and this capacity is coordinated through our nervous system, which when blocked can lead to ill health.

The chiropractic philosophy was firm in me from my mentors, so I decided to go to a less philosophical school thinking that it would be fine. When I say less philosophical I mean pain based, chasing symptoms and doing rehab and physical therapy modalities to try and fix a symptom. This is all fine and well to do, but it just wasn't what I wanted to do. What I really wanted to do was work with kids and generally they don't have pain. They have other things like colic, they spit up, constipation, asthma, allergies, ADD, and autism just to name a few.

So after being at that school for three quarters and feeling unfulfilled in the education I was getting, I decided to transfer to my alma mater Life Chiropractic College West. This school fulfilled me in every way possible. I got an amazing education, had like-minded peers, tons of varying clubs on campus and teachers that knew the chiropractic philosophy and talked about it freely in class. I also had a school president that listened to my plight and let me test out of the classes I had that overlapped in my chiropractic education from Brazil. He is to this day one of my biggest mentors,

Dr. Gerald Clum.

Luckily doing chiropractic school a second time I was able to get the education I really wanted. I deepened my knowledge of how the body works, neurology and really worked on my adjusting skills and got confident with them. I did a diplomate in pediatric chiropractic care, a chiropractic mission trip where we served hundreds of people in a favela in Brazil, traveled around the world through the World Congress of Chiropractic Students, further studied the Upper Cervical techniques I was very interested in. I met many friends and mentors through conferences and gatherings around the US and the globe and then had the pleasure of serving as Valedictorian of my graduating class.

The silver lining was I became a much more confident and competent Doctor of Chiropractic. I widened my network of influential inspiring individuals who mentor me and are my friends to this day. So when you think about quitting something, remember back to why you started. It helps the path become clearer.

Austin Life Chiropractic

2700 W. Anderson Lane, Suite 509

Austin, TX 78757

Phone: (512) 452-7681

Email: juliapinkertondc@gmail.com

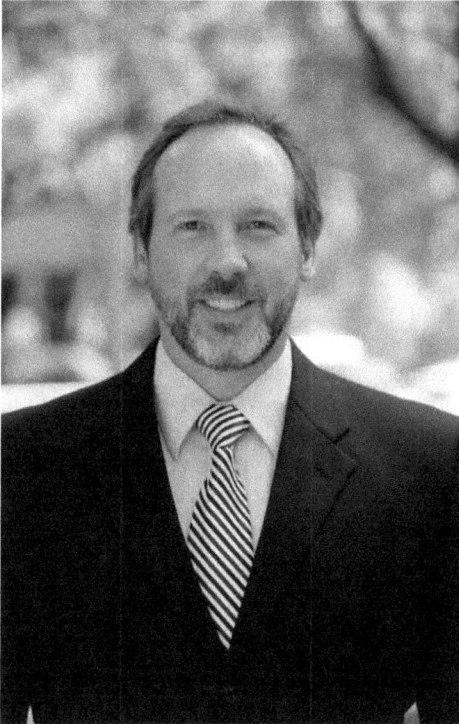

Dr. Mike Hall

"Chiropractic Chose Me"

Southeastern Oklahoma is often referred to as "God's country" by those who reside in the region. Being a young farm boy I knew little of life off the farm and readily accepted my playground of rolling hills, large Oak and Hackberry trees perfect for climbing, ponds that were always ready to receive "hook and line" at a moments' notice, and the chores that began before sunrise and ended with the sunset. I was fortunate to have a father who was very engaged in the development of his young son's endless curiosity and tendencies towards mischief. Once while walking down the road towards the pond I noticed a wet area that seemed to be out of place. I looked to my father to inquire his thoughts. Rather than give me the immediate answer of "looks like a water leak to me", he delayed and instead asked me, "What do you think is the reason for this wet area?" Little did I know at the time that he was quietly forming what was to become my "thought process" for years to come. Only after I had dug a hole and discovered that a rock had worn a hole into the water pipe causing it to leak did my father then show me how to fix this problem. "First thing", he would say to me, "is to identify the cause of the problem and then the fix is easy". How true those words have been in my life and the life of my patients.

High school would come and pass quickly. I graduated at the top of my class and it was time to decide what was to come next? I had performed well in the sciences, so Ms. Williams my guidance counselor set me up to go to medical school. With scholarships and grants I was headed to Oklahoma State University to begin my pre-med studies. That was the plan, simple, right? "Maybe", as Dr. Parker would later tell me, "the universe has a different calling for you." In addition to my school work, I had become an adept cross country runner and miler. In the summer of 1983, while competing at an AAU summer track meet, a mate of mine and I were talking and discussing college and career choices. His mother, Linda, overheard our conversation and asked, "have you ever considered chiropractic?" Reluctantly, I said, "what is chiropractic? I've never heard of it." The cast was being formed.

I decided to check out the local chiropractor at least the closest one in the nearest town. Dr. Ashley had been a chiropractor for 28 years and was well respected in the county. He also had a ranch where he bred prized bulls. After an evaluation, he told me that I had a subluxation in my upper back. I didn't feel bad or hurt. He told me that I might not have any symptoms but as long as there was a vertebrae out of alignment that I couldn't function at my best. As I headed home those words ruminated in my mind over and over. Something about "a vertebrae out of place impairs function" just seemed to make sense to me, really, shouldn't it to everyone.

I looked into the chiropractic colleges and Parker was my choice. I set up a time to visit and check out the campus. When I came to Dallas in the summer of '87, I was directed to a Piggly Wiggly grocery store. I had seen a few of those in other cities. What I didn't realize is that that grocery store was Parker College. It was being renovated for classrooms. So then I was taken over to see the laboratories and gross anatomy lab. Where I was taken was to the church across the street. The basement of the church contained the anatomy lab and the second floor the other labs for various classes. I said to myself, "class in the grocery store and labs in the church – perfect!"

There I met a professor that still imparts his wisdom on me today even though he is no longer with us. His name, Dr. Eugene Kindley, had his PhD in Neuroscience and was the department head of the Basic Sciences. He also taught Neuroscience I & II along with the labs. One day he told me, "Mike, chiropractic does not yet fully realize the impact that the chiropractic adjustment has on the human nervous system." These words rolled over and over in my mind. A mind that was shaped early on to "look for the cause of the problem and the fix would be easy". The question was set, - "How does the subluxation influence the health of an individual?" My purpose in this profession was becoming more and more clear. I continued my studies, excelling in the sciences and adjusting skill sets. I studied with a voracious appetite the neurology of the articulations, the physiology of the neural impulse, and development of the higher centers. Behaviours, thoughts, decision making, as well as chronic pain, depression, and fatigue began to really drive my studies.

The time for graduation was upon me. It was becoming more and more apparent that a part of me was built for teaching others while a part of me was destined to be in the field practicing the art of chiropractic. Upon graduating I was offered an opportunity to become a junior faculty in the Basic Sciences. I opened a clinic and accepted the teaching position as well at Parker College. In clinical practice many of my patients were afflicted with neurological disorders that had up to this point been refractory to traditional treatment applications. Some of those conditions were stroke, cerebral palsy, neuropathy, epilepsy, multiple sclerosis, and the like. It became natural for me to share my clinical experiences in the classroom and soon there was quite an excitement amongst the students for learning neurology. A class that was typically dreaded by most was now being looked forward to as the class "that puts it all together". I went on to complete my post graduate studies in neurology, rehabilitation, and orthopedics. While the certificates and such were not the goal, learning was. I could not learn enough about the subluxation. During this time, the 90's were considered the "decade of the brain" in the research arena. There was much to learn and apply. It was a great time to be a chiropractor!

The 2000's were just as exciting and known as the "decade of cognitive sciences". It would be soon in the Fall of 2009, that a former student, Dr. Francis Murphy, and I would be re-united. It wasn't uncommon to see your former students out in the field, busy with their practices, taking seminars and conferences. It just so happened that I was in Rome preparing to give a presentation for Parker Seminars when Dr. Murphy approached me and was adamant that I see something he had brought. Reluctantly, I agreed and we retreated to a laptop computer to watch a DVD of some case studies. These were amazing videos of patients with "frozen shoulder" being treated with a specialized technique and getting phenomenal results! A bond was formed and we hit the streets to teach other chiropractors!

OTZ was founded and Dr. Murphy and I began travelling across the United States and Europe giving seminars and presentations on this technique. We have presented research, given instruction, and discussed the neurology behind this application to thousands of chiropractors. Research interests have budded, practices have been enhanced, and lives forever changed. What started out as a "frozen shoulder" treatment turned out to be an approach that would change the outcomes of many other conditions from Bell's palsy, autism, ADD/ADHD, to aspects of aphasia and apraxia. Now, not only did chiropractors learn the technique but also learned the "why" in what we are doing. This added a new dimension to the teaching side of the coin in our seminars. Alongside of this technique has been the growth of functional neurology of which I've been practicing for the past 25 years. The degree to which the nervous system can be influenced using environmental cues, neuromuscular activation patterns, and emerging technologies along with innovative applications of neuroscience has given many patients a new hope in life.

My journey in chiropractic has been amazing and filled with countless memories, wonderful mentors, and personal growth. Taking this wonderful healing art to so many patients, in so many places, and changing so many lives has been transformational for me. Coming from such a strong scientific background at a time when chiropractic was struggling for answers to the effects of an adjustment to now seeing the research validate and support chiropractic for its' effects on the brain and body. It is absolutely a paradigm shift in only a relatively few short years. There is still so much work to do but we are off to a great start and the possibilities are energizing. In the neurology world we might say that the prefrontal cortex is being pruned for a whole new synaptic experience! From the early teachings of my father, the influences of teaching faculty and colleagues, caring mentors, training in neurology, practice experiences, and the Parker Principles – I can truly say that "chiropractic chose me" and I'm happy to serve this great profession!

Hall Chiropractic & Neurology Center

215 S. Denton Tap Rd, Suite 285

Coppell, TX 75019

Phone: (972) 304-3900

Fax: (972) 304-2066

www.HallChiropracticWellnessCenter.com

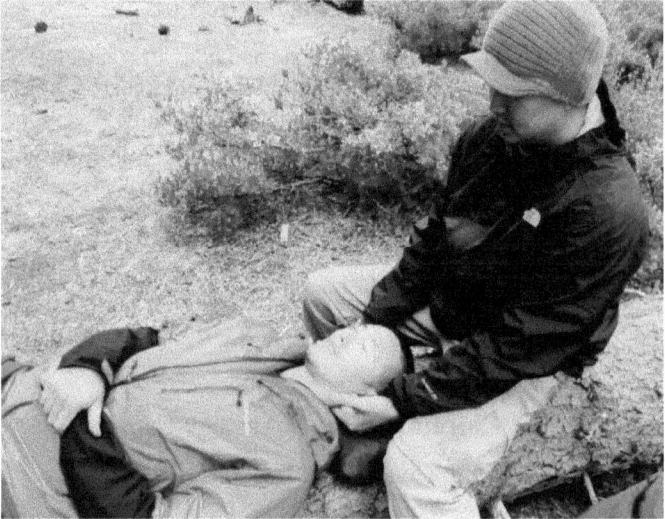

Dr. Stanton Hom

"... Help Others and Serve the World."

"The doctor of the future will give no medicine, but will interest his patients in the care of the human frame, diet and in the cause and prevention of disease."— Thomas A. Edison (1902)

I had just landed in Kuwait when my brother graduated from the Los Angeles College of Chiropractic in April 2003. I deployed as the Battalion Fire Direction Officer for the 4th Battalion 42nd Field Artillery Regiment, 4th Infantry Division and admittedly was also thinking about where my path was taking me. Was I going to stay in the military and carry on my service to our great nation? Or was I going to hang up my uniform and serve the world as a civilian?

The best thing about our deployment was the soldiers we served alongside. 4-42 wasn't your typical artillery battalion. Across the board we were above and beyond the rest of the division artillery. We excelled in every competition, we excelled in combat keeping the city of Ad Dawr safe in Iraq, and we couldn't be touched on the Frisbee Football Field! But as I mentioned above, nothing topped the soldiers and officers.

To this day I miss the camaraderie, the friendships, and I miss knowing that I could trust the guy on my left and right, to get my back at a moment's notice.

While I was deployed, my brother sent me three books to read. The first was "The Web that Has no Weaver by Dr. Ted Kapchuk, the second "Total Health Nutrition" by Dr. Joe Mercola and the last was "Applied Kinesiology" by Dr. Robert Frost. These books were meant to shine a light on a potential new path for me. What I didn't realize was that my brother was slowly becoming the "Doctor of the Future". What I did realize was that he was more inspired and driven than most of our friends and peers. What I could feel in my heart was how strong his purpose was to help others and serve the world.

It made me proud... of him of course, but also of the fact that people like him existed in the world. When you are fighting for the values of this country, when you are laying your life on the line in the name of freedom, you want to know there are people out there serving in a way that has incredible value for the world.

As I read the books, it was as if a veil that I didn't even know existed was lifting. These men wrote about healing from the inside out. They talked about how healing has been a part of our species for 1000s of years and how we didn't need to be filled with drugs to 'cure' every disease. Each of them talked about food as medicine and how in healing less is more.

When I redeployed to Fort Hood, TX, I immediately changed my nutrition to a whole food diet. I thought about not only the number of calories I ate but also the quality of calories I ate. In fact, I was the chef in the house so I became the food dictator for not only myself and also my three roommates. Back then, living in central Texas, there weren't a lot of healthy food options and if you said the word 'organic' people didn't think you were talking about food! But being an hour north of Austin, I bought an ice chest and drove to Whole Foods Market every weekend for our produce.

You see, I couldn't unlearn what I had learned. My mindset around health was changing and I started to realize our choices mattered. As much as my roommates disapproved of spending more on food, they couldn't deny how different our food looked and tasted. They couldn't deny how much better they felt.

When it came time to leave the service, I was still unsure about what I wanted to do. Big companies were headhunting West Point graduates, most of my peers were vying for and earning spots at the top Ivy league business schools in the nation but I could not get 'health' off my mind. In the end, I decided to move to San Diego to learn from my best friend and mentor. Much to the chagrin of my superior officers, I was moving to San Diego to 'find my path' and a few weeks later, I packed up my trusty Nissan Pathfinder and headed West.

Moving to San Diego was an incredible decision. It was like paradise everyday. Saying hello to the beach and the surf and saying goodbye to uniforms and deployments brought new opportunities. The money I saved from my deployment was about to pay off big time as I moved in with my brother and made my first appointment at his office.

What he taught me in those first few weeks was life changing. It brought what I had read in those books to life. He told me I was one of the fittest patients he had. But he was clear that 'fitness' and 'strength' was not synonymous with 'health' and 'well-being'. Steve identified inflammatory patterns that affected my digestion. He taught me that my gut was connected to my nervous system, my immune health and my mental well-being. He noticed how these patterns were affecting my emotions and sleep. He then tied these all back to my nervous system and posture.

Steve showed me yoga, he introduced me to meditation, maybe most importantly he drove me to the beach to buy my first surfboard. I made a choice not to choose a career until I knew more about this new sense of wellness. I needed to learn from experience and make the most of this critical time transitioning to the civilian world. About 6 weeks into care, I was getting adjusted 2-3 times a week and really starting to feel reconnected to 'myself'. At this time, Steve suggested I do the Standard Process Purification Program and although I was already discovering the true meaning of health, it wasn't until I completed the cleanse that I felt like my life had hit the reset button. For those people my age, there is a distinct feeling when you push that reset button on a gaming system - it was like that.

When you clear the body of toxins and create improved spinal and neural health through chiropractic adjustments, we are more likely to realize the incredible potential in the body.

If I sit and think about it, I can FEEL it all over again. I am still in the beginning stages of my practice and I love every moment of everyday because in each moment with each patient there is a potential to give to others what my brother gave to me. It's an incredibly personal mission for us.

While my brother was going to chiropractic school, our grandfather passed away. I was training at the National Training Center at Fort Irwin, California when we got the call over the radio. One of the last times I visited him, he was so weak and he barely remembered us. This man fought in World War II. He and his brother did 100 pushups a day until they were in their 80s. I remember him as if he was a VIP as he walked us down the street in Chinatown (LA). When they did his autopsy, they found cancer all over his body and I remember thinking "How could they just find cancer all over his body?" I know this motivated Steve to serve more. I know it spoke to an inside part of him that the end of our grandfather's life could have had a different ending and I know it helped him begin the process of helping the rest of our family.

Soon after I finished chiropractic school, our grandmother passed away. She was the matriarch of our family and losing her was so hard on all of us. I remember driving up from San Diego multiple times a week to see her. I remember my aunt spending 24 hours a day by her side and my parents making meals for my aunt and giving her a break as much as they could. I remember the day that my grandma met my newborn nephew Kai. I remember how in a blink of an eye, she lit up like a candle. She couldn't speak but we all knew that she knew it was her newest great grandbaby - our newest family member.

I remember one day asking my aunt and the nurse tending to my grandmother if we could feed my grandmother fresh juice or smoothies. The nurse looked at me funny and said 'we don't know what it will do to her'. Watching her reconnect her feeding tube and the 'liquid diet' she was on I decided to look at the label and notice all the 'chemicals' in the pseudofood and ask, "What if we drank this?" The nurse looked at me and said, 'I am not going to drink THAT'. I asked 'why not?' and she said "It will probably make us sick." I then asked, "Why would you feed it to a dying person?" She paused and said, "I... don't know."

That was a cathartic moment that has fueled my life and my practice since. Both my brother and I have been able to help not only our parents and their generation in our family live more healthfully, but Steve and his wife Rachel are raising their family in ways that focus on prevention and holistic well-being.

My practice sees whole families - from newborns to expecting moms to grandparents alike. My practice wants to influence generations to be conscious about their health. Being in a Navy town (Go Army, Beat Navy!), I feel fortunate to help these men and women especially those who are deploying overseas and into harm's way. I love knowing that what I know now is helping curb their experience of chronic stress, digestive problems, subluxation patterns and PTSD. With prevention and a vitalistic approach to health, I love helping my patients need all doctors less - including me.

I love being that Doctor of the Future.

Dr. Stanton Hom

3355 4th Ave.

San Diego, CA 92103

Phone: (619) 458-9491

Email: drstanhom@gmail.com

www.drstantonhom.com

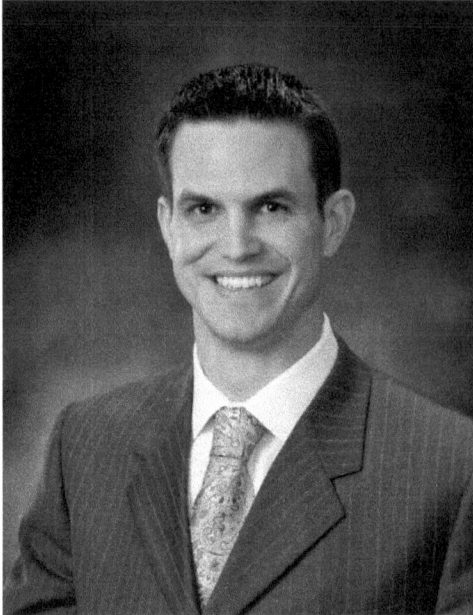

Dr. Vince Scheffler
"... It's My Job..."

Growing up, sports was the main attraction. Whether we were playing them or watching them on TV, it was the glue that kept my family stuck together. That appetite for sports carried over into college where I was fortunate enough to have the ability to play football and get an education.

It was my junior year at Hope College and I was going into the upcoming football season as a preseason All-American. I was studying kinesiology, but did not know what I wanted to actually do with the rest of my life. All I know is that it had to include something with sports.

I had everything going for me, and then it happened… an injury that would lay the framework for the rest of my life. As a punter on the football team, your single most important muscle is your hamstring and I had strained it severely. I went through the conventional treatment forms and had minimal relief. I had multiple shots and took pills and nothing seemed to alleviate the pain. An MRI showed I had torn the hamstring moderately at its insertion on the bone. While it was not an injury that would prevent me from living, it was one that would prevent me from doing the thing I loved most… playing sports.

By midseason I was playing through the injury but it was definitely altering my performance and my mood. One day at practice a friend of mine on the team came up to me and said, "Why don't you go see my dad and see if he can help you?" I asked my friend, what does your dad do? He said, "He is a chiropractor."

There must've been a very long pause at this point in the conversation because I remember going through my head as to why a chiropractor would be able to help me with this injury. Somehow these words that I was thinking in my head came out and were spoken. My friend specifically told me how aligning my pelvis and releasing the muscle in the affected area could greatly help the area heal.

At this point I was up for anything because I was desperate to feel better and most importantly play better. I drove 30 minutes to his dad's office and received my first treatment. He executed the treatment and I remember thinking once he aligned my pelvis… That's it? He then did some myofascial release to my hamstring which was not the most pleasant thing in the world, but I got through it. I didn't know if it was in my head because I wanted to feel better, but I actually felt improvement immediately after getting up off of his table. On the way home, I kept stretching the muscle in a specific way that always hurt me and it continued to be dramatically less. I thought maybe there is something to this. I went back again for multiple treatments over the next couple weeks and each time the pain lessened. I couldn't believe all the pain and stress that I had gone through was gone so simply, after just a few treatments. The even crazier thing in my head was how it all made so much sense to me as to why my pain was gone.

That following spring I had to do an internship for my major, and I decided that I would do it at Dr. Wilcox's office. I watched people walk in incredible amounts of pain and walk out so happy having their pain diminished greatly or removed completely. I was continually amazed. I quickly realized that this was what I wanted to do with the rest of my life.

I attended chiropractic school at Parker university in Dallas, Texas and was offered a job by a local sports chiropractor before I even graduated. During my time there I traveled all over the world treating athletes of all types. From multiple Olympic gold medalist to world class cyclists to the greatest football players in the world, I have been blessed beyond words to do what I love. I now practice back in Michigan working with that same football team that started it all for me.

As I approach my 10th year in practice there are 2 constants that reign supreme no matter where I am. People are people and motion is life. We all have a game to play, and it's my job to make sure that you never miss a second of the action.

Chiropractic Unlimited

5060 Cascade Rd. Suite E

Grand Rapids, MI 49546

Phone: (616) 940-4647

www.chirounlimited.com

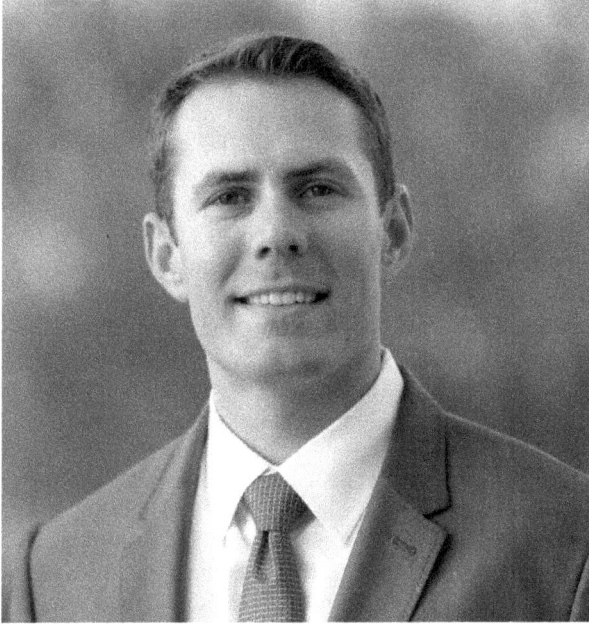

Dr. Lance Cohen, D.C.

"Being in Service"

My chiropractic story began when I was 5 years old, for that is when I formed my first memories and developed my initial understanding of chiropractic. My father, Dr. Nathan Cohen, graduated from the Los Angeles campus of Cleveland Chiropractic College in December of 1980. As time would tell, I would graduate Salutatorian of my class from this same institution 30 years later. Back to the beginning, as a young boy I remember my father helping his patients with debilitating pain or problems. I saw how grateful the people were to receive relief through this non-invasive natural approach. That is when something clicked in my head and a little voice inside me said this is what I want to do when I grow up. I grew up living in a chiropractic family and living the chiropractic lifestyle. My mother received chiropractic adjustments throughout her pregnancy and I began receiving adjustments soon after birth. In addition to regular adjustments, diet, nutrition, physical activity, and positive thinking were all important parts of my childhood. I was always the kid at school with the "gross food" in my lunch, homemade zucchini bread, carob pudding instead of chocolate, rice milk instead of Capri Sun. Most kids enjoyed their Lunchables, Kool Aid, Doritos and Oreos, while I was unappreciatively and reluctantly eating my homemade and health food store bought cuisine. At the time I thought, "What did I do to deserve this from my parents," and to make matters worse I was teased and ridiculed by my peers for what my parents packed in my lunch pail. It wasn't until my late teens to early twenties that I began to appreciate the lifestyle and diet that my parents imposed upon me. Looking back, I didn't have acne; I didn't break any bones, or have any allergies, asthma, or any other significant health problems during my formative years.

I grew up in the Lake Tahoe Basin partaking in many physical outdoor activities and sports. In junior high and high school I played ice hockey, competed in alpine and cross-country skiing, raced sailboats, wake boarded, water-skied, competed in mountain bike racing, camped and backpacked throughout my rugged mountainous surroundings. Throughout all of these competitive and recreational activities I know that the regular chiropractic care my father provided me, kept me in the game, helped move me closer to the podium, or help put me back together after an injury. Likewise, while competing in sports I learned very quickly how important putting the right fuel in your body prior to training or a competition is.

From the time I was able to understand the concept of chiropractic until the summer before I began chiropractic college I had formed my idea of what chiropractic was. I had done so by piecing together observations of my father's practice, his colleagues, and all the information I had soaked up during all the chiropractic seminars that I was dragged to. Some of the seminars were not that bad such as weeklong continuing education on the island of Maui.

So when I showed up for the first day at a chiropractic college to take advantage of the legacy scholarship that they offered me, I thought I had a pretty good idea of what I had signed up for. Boy was I naive.

I vividly remember being overwhelmed in my first gross anatomy class. Just learning the details and parts of a single vertebra was a challenge. Soon after that we were immersed in histology, immunology, pathology, radiology and the rest of the 'ology' alphabet soup. My head was spinning; I had no idea I would be expected to master all these topics of study. Right from the beginning we had chiropractic skills training labs, which were hands on, where I excelled in these classes even though they were challenging.

I applied myself more in chiropractic college than I had ever done so in my student career. I really enjoyed what I was studying and was motivated by the fact that the health of my future patients was at stake. I excelled in the program receiving several merit-based scholarships, receiving the highest scores on my national board's part one and part two at my college, and taking on leadership roles in several student organizations at my college and even on a national and international level. Throughout all of this I continued to excel, to build a network of connections and relationships with influential people in the profession and do everything I could to contribute to the greater good.

Somewhere along the line I found out about a very exclusive internship program with Dr. William Morgan at the National Naval Medical Center (NNMC) in Bethesda, Maryland (now Walter Reed National Military Medical Center). No student from our campus had ever participated in the program. I remember speaking to our college president, dean and clinic director expressing that our college should participate in programs like this if the college aspired to offer a top notch education. That was the beginning of a lot of hard work by many people, but eventually our college signed a memorandum of understanding with the United States Navy which opened the door for students from our college to at least apply for the sought after internship. I hadn't really thought about applying for the program since I had planned to work for my father after graduation and our campus required that our entire clinical requirement be completed at the college clinic prior to any off campus internships. One day our clinic director called me into his office and asked me if I would like to apply for the position. I didn't really think it would work out with my schedule but after some encouragement he convinced me to apply. I set my sights on the internship and began strategizing and forming a plan to position myself as the most eligible candidate. I even made arrangements to meet with Dr. Morgan and tour the medical center.

I wrote down my goals, set my mind to it and worked hard to achieve the action steps in order to be selected for the internship. The hard work paid huge dividends. I will never forget how surprised I was to receive the call from Dr. Morgan offering me the position. It was to be a three-month chiropractic internship and a three-month postdoctoral fellowship in integrated medicine. I would prove to be only the second chiropractor ever to complete this fellowship. The 6 months I spent at NNMC were the most high yield experience of my education. I learned more about chiropractic, patient care and the allopathic model of medicine than I could have ever imagined. Not to mention the lessons of sacrifice, courage, and numerous other qualities I learned from the patients with whom I had the pleasure of interacting and providing care to. Three days a week I adjusted patients in the chiropractic clinic and the other two days a week I rotated through the other services in the hospital. I also had the pleasure of aiding Dr. Morgan in providing chiropractic care to the United States Naval Academy athletes, including their football players and was invited to provide chiropractic services at Camp David.

My time in Bethesda was comprised of amazing experiences that furthered my knowledge as a doctor, expanded my compassion for my fellow man, and opened my eyes to the atrocities of war as well as to the sacrifice of the brave men and women who answer the call to defend our country and our freedom. I also learned about the sacrifices their families make. I departed from Bethesda having made some lifelong friends, in both the staff and the patients.

Transitioning from the hospital to join my father's private practice in La Jolla, California, provided me with new challenges. I quickly learned the differences between one of the largest tertiary care hospitals in the world with over 5000 employees and small business. I was getting a crash course in entrepreneurship; learning things about budgets, logistics, banking, payroll utilities, lease negotiation, marketing, inventory, billing and human resources. These were a lot of topics that were somehow neglected during my combined 9 years of college education.

I have been in private practice with my father for over 5 years; there have been many challenges and obstacles to overcome. Several years ago I purchased my own practice and now split my time between that office and my father's practice. Between the two of us we have three offices and are continuing to grow.

My story does not end here. Many people have experienced profound results from chiropractic, how chiropractic miraculously gave them their lives back and as a result they dedicated their lives to the profession in order to help others in the way that they were once helped by a doctor of chiropractic. During my life I have seen and experienced lots of great results from chiropractic, but that is all I have ever known, it's what I grew up with.

I had to wait until the age of 31 to receive my chiropractic miracle. I was performing an exercise, one which I had recommended for many of my patients, a plank. That is when I felt something happen in my low back that didn't feel right. I stood up and had back pain that traveled down both of my legs and went all the way to my feet. Over the next hours and days it only got worse. The pain was like no other back pain I had ever experienced and I was scared because I could hardly walk. I was in so much pain that I didn't think I could even tolerate an adjustment; however, a good friend of mine, another second-generation chiropractor, talked me into letting him take a look at me.

I felt some immediate improvement after the first adjustment and my left Achilles reflex improved notably. I visited him the next two days for more adjustments. By the fourth day about 90 percent of my pain had resolved and I regained almost all of the function in my legs. I was feeling much better but still wanted to find out what had caused this unusual episode. So with the help of a medical doctor, I utilized my health insurance for the first time and had a full medical work up to include new blood tests, new X-rays and finally an MRI. The MRI revealed a substantially large tumor taking up about 80 percent of my spinal canal at L1. The tumor was compressing all the nerves that went to my lower extremities. I was shocked to say the least, for I believed I was in great health and yet in front of my eyes was something I never expected. What I found equally amazing was in the course of three spinal adjustments over four days my symptoms improved so significantly. This was truly a chiropractic miracle. The adjustments didn't cure me of my tumor but they took my pain from a 7/10 to a 1/10 and allowed me to walk and perform the activities of daily living for several months until I was able to have neurosurgery in order to remove the tumor.

While writing this story I am four weeks post surgery. I was fortunate to have one of the top neurosurgeons in the world, one of only a handful of surgeons who perform the type of surgery I needed in a minimally invasive approach. He did an amazing job and at my three week follow up he told me that I am a model patient and I am healing very quickly.

My training as a doctor of chiropractic and my understanding of the spine and nervous system drove me to seek out a surgeon who could remove this tumor while sparing as much of the spine and surrounding tissues as possible. It was also my training as a doctor of chiropractic that guided me to eat right, think right, and move right after the surgery to ensure a speedy recovery.

Cohen Chiropractic Clinic

8813 Villa La Jolla Drive

Suite 2010

La Jolla, CA 92037

855-61-CHIRO (24476)

www.cohenchiroclinic.com

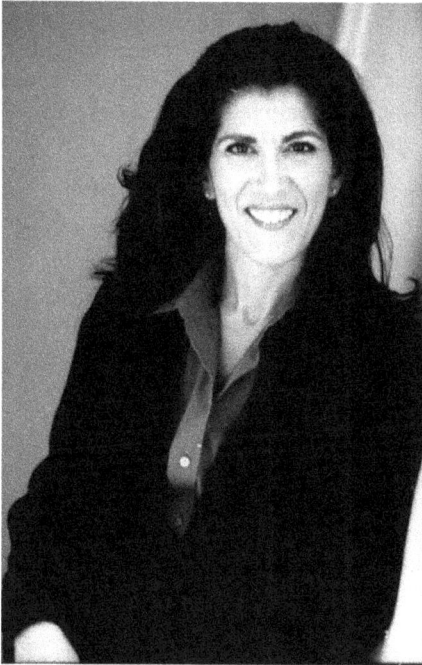

Dr. Carol Ann Malizia, D.C.

"Chiropractic: A Family Tradition"

No greater gift was ever given to me than the ability to make a difference and create hope in another. Being "in service" through the power of chiropractic was never a job to me. It was a calling.

Throughout my career, I learned that being in service and loving what I do meant that I never had to work a day in my life – the realization of something my father would always tell me when I was growing up.

Raised at the United States Military Academy, I've been immersed in the traditions of the Long Grey Line at West Point since before I was born. I always teased my parents that the music of the Washington Post March stirred something in me every time I heard it – whether I was in the band in elementary school and high school, or even later in my adult life – just because I heard it nearly every day while my mother was pregnant with me at West Point.

My father, my greatest buddy and mentor, was the captain of the percussion section for the United States Military Band at that time, so I grew up with a strong kinesthetic love of vibration from all the instruments we had in our basement: Kettle drums, xylophones, standing chimes, snare drums, field drums – everything and anything that was dependent on vibration and eye-hand coordination to make sound. Looking back now, I am fascinated how my early recollections of structure, function and tone may have in fact formed the foundation for my career as a chiropractor.

My father took me for my first chiropractic adjustment when I was around 10 years old. He had gotten the "big idea" about chiropractic many years before, so I grew up with regular chiropractic visits due to his influence.

One thing that is apparent when you live in the United States Military Academy is that there is no shortage of structure and function. From the arrangement of the vast buildings to the landscape of the base – which is mostly uphill if you speak to a new cadet – to the academic curriculum, all the systems are built on discipline, precision, and "Duty, Honor and Country." Watching the educational strategies, "plebe knowledge," sports, marching formations and mess hall feedings (20 minutes to feed 2,000 cadets, three times per day), you get the sense that there are a lot of systems operating around you.

The same can be said of the human body, and my experience growing up repeated itself as I learned about our biological systems and organization while studying for a career in chiropractic. I was fascinated at how the body kept up with all the systems through the influence and the control of the nervous system. Equally as captivating to me was the ability to communicate with the body from the outside, especially after it was compromised by a stressor – structurally, chemically, or mentally/emotionally from a trauma.

The most amazing sensation would emerge as I learned to detect areas of the spine that were out of alignment. Even more incredible was when I removed the subluxation, or interference, in the system. The structures were not only restored, but the patients would report circumstances, functions and healings that were ALL about their bodies healing themselves. I was merely the facilitator.

One day, there was a little girl with beautiful red hair in my reception room, leaning into her mother with her blanket tucked under her chin and clutching her favorite stuffed animal, which my terrific staff had advised her to bring so we could check its spine as well. She had dark circles under her eyes and a white, drawn in complexion covered with cracked, bleeding, oozing red patches. My heart nearly fell out when I walked into the new patient exam and saw this child, and I could feel her mother's anguish, pain and sleepless nights the moment I entered the room. We did a history and examination, and got right to work. She'd had no bowel movements, no appetite, no sleep, and wasn't playing with her siblings – she was just miserable. Freeing her spine of interference was like bringing the communication back into her circuit boards. I made sure to tell my little beauty she was going to hear some popcorn and that everything was going to be alright.

When I lifted her off the table after her adjustment, I looked into her eyes and she immediately smiled back at me, got her stuffed animal and put its head in the proper position on my adjusting table. Her mother and I shared a brief glance with tears in both of our eyes, and then I showed her how to help her toy's spine. I advised the mother on some whole food nutrients and menu modifications, scheduled a follow-up after the weekend on Monday, plus three more visits over the next week.

The following Friday, I was helping an elderly patient through the reception room, and in the corner caught my eye was a child sitting with a pile of stuffed animals on her lap. When I ran back through the reception room door they were already in one of the adjusting rooms, so I could not immediately see who it was.

I was in such disbelief – I had run right by my little beauty, now sitting with at least ten stuffed animals, all waiting to get their spines checked! I didn't even recognize her as the same child as the week before! She was radiant, chatting, smiling and laughing, without a blemish or a crack in her complexion, and no evidence of oozing from her arms, legs or face! I shake my head now, fully remembering that little girl and knowing in my heart that everyone deserves the moment where structure corrects function.

The impact of chiropractic on the hundreds of patients I saw looked different in every case, and in many cases they taught me profound life lessons – often in the most humbling of circumstances.

Fifteen years ago, I walked into a room with a family waiting for their adjustments – not uncommon to see at 4:30 on a busy weekday afternoon – and chose to ignore my gut feeling that the energy was off in the room. The mother made the request to adjust the two children first; she would go last and then she needed to talk to me, confirming my gut feeling that something was wrong.

When someone makes such a request coming from a busy reception room, you start to brace yourself for impact. However, I was not even remotely prepared for what was about to be revealed. You see, her husband had just been pulled out of the Hudson River after a drowning accident, and they had to go to the hospital to identify the body. The mother had read that adjustments can impact emotional health, and her hope was that it may help her children cope with the devastating news and situation if they were adjusted first. The shock in the room was palpable. After all she was going through, my office was the first place she called.

Structure can correct function.

To this day, I have no idea how I went into the next room to adjust the next patient after making every attempt to control my emotions for this family.

Many years later, I was giving a presentation in Atlanta to a room of nearly 200 chiropractic assistants. At that time, most CAs were women, so I was surprised to see a tall, handsome young man fill the door frame at the back of the room. As he came toward me and started to speak, I noticed that he had a very familiar voice. It was the woman's son! With a huge hug, he lifted me off my feet and told me he had just graduated chiropractic school.

"Dr. Carol Ann," he said. "I just wanted you to know how much I love being a Chiropractor! Do you remember adjusting me the day my Dad passed? It had such an impression on me that I decided to become one just like you!"

Again, structure correcting function.

In recent years, there was a shift in my service. My sister was part of a unique group of women leaders that found a place in history as part of the first generation of women at West Point. One of her classmates was retired Brigadier General Rebecca Halstead, who I met while she was doing a keynote presentation in the Cadet Mess Hall at West Point, and that day has come to shape a new meaning of being "in service" for me.

Of the 600 people in attendance that day, the woman that had sat next to me for the keynote presentation was chatting with me about how her daughter was raised with chiropractic care and was a strong advocate, but unfortunately she no longer had access to it. Naturally, I asked who her daughter was and where she lived, hoping to find her a good referral.

The woman pointed to Rebecca and said, "That's my daughter, and she lives in Iraq! She's suffering with horrible, chronic fibromyalgia."

As the mother asked if I would be willing to check her daughter before she left that day, I heard my father's voice in my head saying, "Sweetheart, with knowledge comes responsibility."

From that day forward, and for the last 6 years, we have diligently worked with the structure and function of one of our nation's bravest, most courageous and most passionate soldiers. After three years, she was off all 16 medications she had been taking; thriving in life rather than just surviving, with a life goal of helping others that she knew were suffering as once she had.

Service all comes down to duty, honor and country, much like the motto and creed of West Point.

We have a duty to each and every person we meet, to teach them how to honor their own body's ability to adapt and heal so that we can help them elevate their quality of life, along with the potential to maximize their own structure and function.

In chiropractic and in my career, I have learned that being in service to my country does not require a uniform. I will always be armed with hope, and in service to those who have served in our military.

Dr. Carol Ann Malizia

Doctor of Chiropractic

CAM Integrated Consulting

Newburgh, New York 12550

Email: camdc63@aol.com

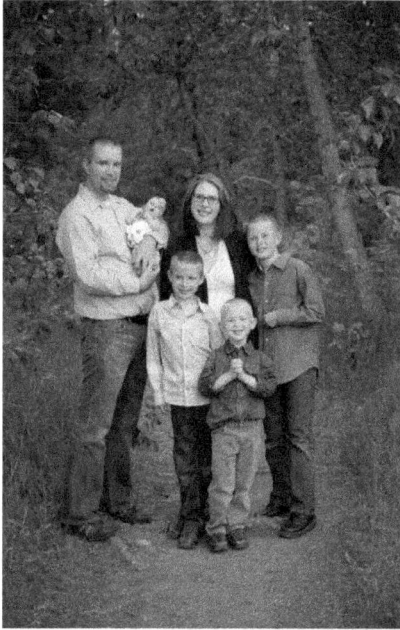

Dr. Katherine A. Pohlman

D.C., PhD, D.I.C.C.P.

"... Healthcare our Family Enjoys..."

I was originally drawn to a career in chiropractic because of its emphasis on non-invasive care, concentration on the patient's overall health, and the uniqueness of the chiropractor doctor-patient relationship. Throughout my training at Palmer College of Chiropractic, I was intrigued by both the emphasis on development of the doctor-patient relationship as well as chiropractic care for the pediatric and pregnant population. However, I frequently ended up with more questions at the end of the day than I had at the beginning. During my clinical internship, these questions became even more relevant. It was not uncommon to see a patient have a rapid, positive response to chiropractic care and then, the next week, a patient who appeared to have a similar presentation not respond to what seemed to me to be a very similar treatment. Trying to find answers to questions of this nature drew me to the chiropractic research literature; thus I began to identify the many knowledge gaps that needed to be filled in order to help me and other chiropractic clinicians provide the very best quality patient care possible. This led me to apply to the Master's in Clinical Research program at Palmer College.

During my first year in the Master's (MS) program, I worked as a Study Coordinator in the research clinic. This role matched my interest in how chiropractic care impacts patient's outcomes and my skill in attention to detail. Through my coursework and work efforts I quickly gained an even greater appreciation for the importance of and need for research in the chiropractic profession, particularly for children. I was surrounded by mentors that had the same passion, commitment, and dedication that I felt and realized that I too could make a difference. Thus, my vision of becoming a chiropractic scientist solidified.

After completing my first year in the Clinical Research Master's program (2007), I was invited to apply for a clinical project manager (CPM) job position open at the Palmer Center for Chiropractic Research (PCCR). The position called for someone able to manage multiple externally funded clinical research projects, acting as the key liaison between the principal investigator, clinic core personnel, and the Office of Data Management and Biostatistics. Since I am avid about organization and detail, and am a proponent of the importance of good communication in teams, this position offered a perfect opportunity to gain more experience conducting research, while still allowing me to complete my Master of Science degree on a part-time basis.

I graduated with my MS degree in 2010 and after 3 productive years in the CPM role for two federally funded clinical trials, I was hired as the Clinical Project Manager II (CPMII) at the PCCR. The CPMII role allows me to continue my successful monitoring and training role, but also gives me an opportunity to be a supervisor and the lead CPM for the Department of Defense (DoD) grant to conduct three distinct clinical trials, one which presents the single largest chiropractic multi-site LBP controlled trial within the chiropractic profession.

Throughout this time period, I was also engaging in pediatric chiropractic research in two ways. In 2007, I became the vice president for the American Chiropractic Association-Council on Chiropractic Pediatrics, a position that I held until 2013. In 2008, I received a clinical chiropractic pediatric certification from the International Clinical Chiropractic Pediatrics by participating in a post-graduate training program. This program is an in-depth clinical experience focused on effective and safe treatment of this population. Instructors of the courses where filled with passion and commitment to bringing the best care for children. Nevertheless, like my chiropractic training, this experience left me with even more questions; thus, I became even more committed to a research career.

My Master's requirement was surrounded around my pediatric chiropractic research interest, conducting two mentored research projects related to this topic. The first project was a job analysis of doctors of chiropractic (DCs) with the same pediatric diplomate certification that I had obtained. The goal was to explore if material taught in the curriculum was actually utilized by practicing DCs. I found that the percentage of pediatric cases seen in these practices was higher than that of US DCs across the country. My second project was to conduct a prospective case series on pregnant females with low back pain in a unique integrative environment in the Appalachian region of Ohio. From this project I gained experience working remotely with health care providers naïve to research protocols.

Following the experiences gained from these two projects, I began looking for additional opportunities within this realm. I learned about a unique PhD opportunity with the Complementary and Alternative Research and Education (CARE) program at the University of Alberta, under the supervision of Drs. Sunita Vohra and Linda Carroll. I applied and was accepted in July, 2011. As part of my training, I have been the lead study coordinator for a Canadian Institutes of Health Research team grant whose goal is to support a patient safety culture for spinal manipulation therapy providers. With this position, I have been honored to have additional mentors who are both international and interdisciplinary content experts. My PhD thesis is titled 'Improving the assessment of safety in pediatric chiropractic manual therapy: a RCT evaluating passive versus active surveillance assessing pediatric adverse events after chiropractic care.'

When my residency requirements were met at the University of Alberta, I wanted to head back to the chiropractic arena. An opportunity was available at Parker University in Dallas, TX as an Assistant Professor, Clinical Research Scientist. With an established Research Institute and enthusiastic administrators and faculty, I knew that joining Parker University would allow me to both continue my own research agenda and help others learn how to apply evidence within their practice.

In parallel with all my career aspirations described above, I have also been blessed with an incredibly supportive husband, who is also a doctor of chiropractic. Together, throughout all my education, we have created a beautiful family, filled with love, laughter, some tears, and lots of joys. Our first son was born in the middle of my chiropractic education, our second son was born when I was in the MS program and a few weeks after my husband graduated as a chiropractor, and our third son was born a few weeks after I graduated with my MS degree. Our final addition, a little girl, arrived during our time in Canada, shortly before our move back to the USA. It is this family, which provides me perspective to balance family and career, as well as the motivation to help open more doors for other families to have the type of healthcare our family enjoys every day.

Katherine A. Pohlman, DC, MS, DICCP

2500 Walnut Hill Lane

Dallas, TX 75229

Phone: (214) 438-6932 ext. 7148

Fax: (214) 902-2482

Email: kpohlman@parker.edu

www.parker.edu

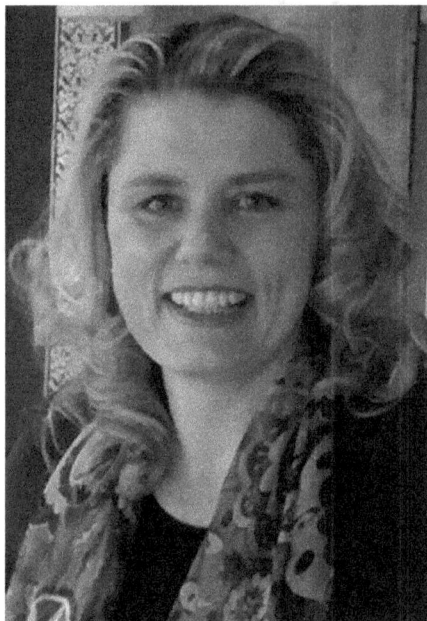

Dr. Sherry McAllister

M.S. (ed.), D.C., C.C.S.P.

"... Peace and Balance..."

I slipped into a pair of brand new riding boots, with a cowboy hat upon my head and ready to test the speed of my feet in a country dance class. In my neighborhood this was the way to spend a Saturday night living in Calgary Alberta, the home of the world famous Calgary Stampede. This was the best way to blow off steam while pursuing a degree in Cellular Molecular Microbial Biology. Many hours looking into a microscope, hauling heavy books back and forth to class and spending countless hours behind the computer reviewing, analyzing and developing conclusions to the experiments performed.

As I headed out that Saturday night little did I know it would change my life forever! The sky was clear, a warm September eve and night for fun and friendship. Just a few short miles to our destination, the driver pulled up to a red light and stopped. Moments later we could both hearing screeching tires behind us. This screeching sound is the sound that you immediately know is not going to be good. We were hit from behind at the red light with extensive impact to the vehicle. Not only could you feel the intense rear impact but felt the car lifting off the ground. Popping sounds, bending metal and breaking glass were all part of the slow motion experience that enveloped our fragile human frames. The next memory was that of a paramedic asking me if I was hurt. My immediate thought was I am okay, however as I started to try to take off the seatbelt I felt numbness and tingling down my right leg and a throbbing sensation in my head. This was the beginning to my new challenges ahead.

The next few months felt like a lifetime. The pain was severe in my head, the numbness in my right leg was beyond frustrating. I recall going to a movie with a friend and getting up from the movie style seats and taking a step on my right foot and almost falling to my knees as I could not feel the bottom of my right foot hitting the ground. The medical doctor prescribed a host of pain killers, anti-inflammatories and physical therapy. I was adamant about getting better so I followed the prescription protocol which made me extremely tired and my stomach beyond upset for the majority of the day. I went to the physical therapist three times a week and remembering that each visit was to add to the last. I was disheartened after several months. I thought that I would need to learn to live with this level of discomfort and may need to change the career path I was on as looking into a microscope created a throbbing, sharp headache that would increase in intensity the longer I continued looking into the microscope.

Six months of pain, medication, depression and desperation led me to try something new. While sitting in a physics class a fellow classmate explained that I should try chiropractic. He reached over and gave me a card to his chiropractor. That afternoon was riddled with uncertainty. I thought, (like most of the patients I see in my office) that if this was a viable choice why didn't my MD send me to one. So I sat in the waiting room anxious and fearful as I didn't want my headaches to get worse.

The chiropractor greeted me with a smile and warmth that I had not ever seen to date during my care. He spent time going through my history like no other. He took x-rays and compared them to the ones taken from the hospital. His explanations were thorough and I immediately felt as if he could truly understand the pain I was experiencing. I had suffered six months of headaches every day, creating difficulty with sleep, concentration, and reading. That afternoon, after my first adjustment, my headache went away!

It was shortly thereafter I began my research on what it would take to become a chiropractor. After finishing my Bachelor's degree I made a choice to go to the chiropractic school that started it all: Palmer College. David Daniel Palmer is the founding father of chiropractic. His work and passion is what created a profession that promotes holistic wellbeing. The history was rich, the research outstanding and instructors were writing books, lecturing internationally and leading the profession. I am so very proud to be a Palmer Alumni.

After graduating from Palmer I realized I could continue to educate those around me on the vitalistic power of the human frame. This prompted me to get my Master's Degree in Science with a focus on Education, allowing opportunities to educate greater audiences. I began teaching at the Chiropractic College as well as the local Junior College by my house while starting my practice.

Opening my own practice has been one of the greatest joys. It has been almost twenty years now in family practice and it has grown so tremendously that I can share the success with three other doctors in my office. Every day I witness the miracles of healing, the patients laughing, and observing them enjoying the benefits that caring for their health can provide. I practice what I preach so you may see me on the marathon trail, running track with my boys or sitting in a seminar to learn more about health.

It's hard to fully appreciate the impact one adjustment can create. I was giving up on being healthy ever again, and believing that painkillers would be a daily regimen. That afternoon changed my life, and ultimately my career aspirations. I wanted to do for others what was done for me. I wanted to provide hope, health, education and a vital understanding that the body is a fascinating complex structure that given the opportunity will heal itself! A famous philosopher: Lao Tzu once said: "When I let go of what I am, I become what I might be." I gave up the structured warfare on bacteria and virus to find peace and balance in the human frame.

McAllister Chiropractic

1645 Willow Street Suite 100

San Jose, CA 95125

Phone: (408) 264-4216

Email: dr.mcallister@sbcglobal.net

www.mcallisterchiro.com

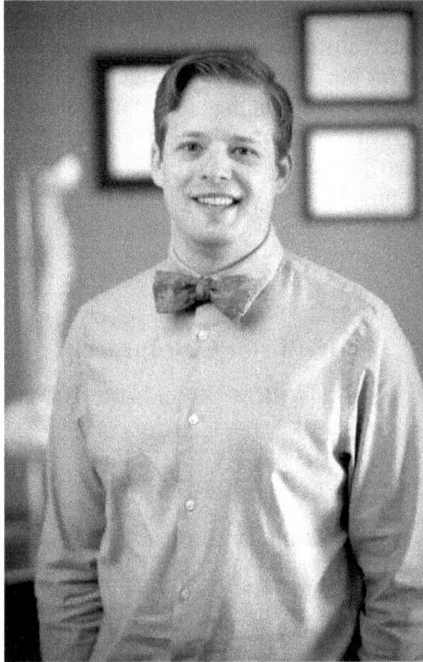

Dr. Eric J. Roseen, D.C.

"... A Very Exciting Field..."

My career began with my experience as a patient. I grew up in rural North Dakota and during my sophomore year of high school, I rolled over my neck at a wrestling tournament. The level of pain was intense; my movement was limited and I was unable to get relief from stretching or over the counter medication. Not being able to compete was a very troubling thing for me, as I was completely dedicated to my sport. I, like many Americans, equated healthcare to seeing a medical physician, and receiving a prescription for a medication to alleviate symptoms. My wrestling coach broadened my healthcare experience by recommending that I go to a chiropractor first.

My chiropractor, Dr. Bonnie Frieje, of Devils Lake, ND assessed me carefully and helped me better understand why I was experiencing pain and how she could help me. I will never forget how effective her care was. In just a few visits I was back to practice as if nothing had happened. Dr. Frieje also identified imbalances in my back, shoulders and neck that I had developed through my sport. She explained that some of my soft tissues were short and tight and others where long and weak. She gave me exercises and stretches to perform to help improve my mechanics and prevent recurrence of pain. I was completely impressed by Dr. Frieje's expertise and fascinated by her hands on approach to healing.

Throughout high school and college I spent time reading about chiropractic and other healthcare professions. I always came back to my personal experience with chiropractic and my interest in anatomy, movement and hands on treatment. Following college, my group of friends spread out across the United States, matriculating at colleges of medicine, osteopathy, physical therapy, and chiropractic. I looked forward to working with my peers and wondered how we could collaborate on patient care.

I moved to Portland, Oregon to study chiropractic at the University of Western States. On my first week of class, I met a lot of likeminded peers with similar reports of positive responses to chiropractic care. Being surrounded by colleagues was inspiring and I was very excited about the impact we would make on the lives of our patients - helping many individuals move past their condition and return to work and activities they love.

In my first year of Chiropractic College, I realized that there were barriers to accessing chiropractic care. Not everyone with musculoskeletal injury will receive a prompt referral to a chiropractor like I had as a wrestler in high school. I was surprised to hear that in the United States less than 10 percent of the public utilizes chiropractic care each year. Chiropractors were inadequately integrated into mainstream healthcare systems and the vast majority of chiropractors worked in private practices. I thought of my college friends who were now working in a wide range of healthcare careers - I again wondered how we could work together to improve care for Americans experiencing common musculoskeletal conditions. I became very interested in the role chiropractors could play within a larger healthcare team, especially in primary care settings.

I became very involved with the Student American Chiropractic Association (SACA) locally and nationally. As the SACA National Vice-Chair I engaged with my peers and leaders of the profession to learn more about the history and future of chiropractic within the US healthcare system. At the 2011 National Chiropractic Legislative Conference (NCLC), we lobbied our nations leaders in Washington D.C. just weeks before the Affordable Care Act (ACA) was passed into law. Participating in the beginnings of healthcare reform was a tremendously inspiring lesson in advocacy and healthcare policy. We were part of history. The experience helped me understand how my generation of chiropractic students could learn to operate in reform of the U.S. healthcare system and advocate for broadened health choices for Americans.

My exposure to the Oregon Collaborative for Integrative Medicine (OCIM) as a student was equally impactful. I was a founding member of a student organization established under the umbrella of the OCIM, which we called the Student Alliance for Integrative Medicine (SAIM). SAIM brought together motivated, collaborative and altruistic students of chiropractic, naturopathy, osteopathy, allopathic and traditional Chinese medicine. It was impressed upon us that this experience of learning together was very rare, which is unfortunate. We were excited to understand our differences, similarities, strengths and 'languages'. It took effort and time to start to understand potential opportunities for collaborating clinically. I learned how acupuncture, massage and medication could benefit my future patients. I believe that through exploring these large knowledge gaps with my future colleagues we became better, more patient centered providers.

I moved to Massachusetts to do an internship at a hospital-based spine center. With a chiropractor as the medical director of this center, this multidisciplinary team took an evidence-based approach to the management of back pain. I fell in love with the academic fervor of Boston and wanted to stay in this healthcare mecca. After graduation, I worked at a primary care center in Dedham, MA. I was part of a large team including medical doctors, acupuncturists, physical therapists, massage therapists, and dieticians. I regularly attended lectures at the many academic instructions in Boston, developing relationships through my curiosity about the complexity of healthcare systems.

I really enjoy working with athletes, especially runners. I've worked with runners at the Boston Marathon since moving to the city. I recently moved my practice to a multidisciplinary clinic in Boston's Kenmore Square, blocks away from Fenway Park, the stadium of the Red Sox. Here I work closely with a team of providers to help patients recover from injury and return to the activities they love.

It is my long-term goal to become a clinician researcher. To help chiropractors and other healthcare providers better understand musculoskeletal conditions and improve outcomes for the patients we serve. I'm currently a Research Fellow in the Family Medicine Department at Boston University and Boston Medical Center. I met my research mentor, Rob Saper MD MPH, after attending a lecture at one of Boston's academic hospitals. Dr. Saper's research is focused on yoga for chronic low back pain in low-income ethnically-diverse primary care populations. I was impressed with his work and interest in the tremendous impact of back pain on society. Our mutual interests fueled the writing of a grant that currently funds my fellowship. The National Institute of Health (NIH) National Center for Complementary and Integrative Health has a number of grants that are available to encourage early-career doctors of chiropractic, and other integrative medicine providers, to gain research skills through research experiences. As a Fellow I've worked on multiple ongoing clinical trials, I am completing a MS degree in Epidemiology and have the opportunity to interact and learn from a wide range of clinicians and researchers.

I am fortunate to have found my wife along my journey so far. She is beginning a career in general medicine and it has been wonderful to learn from each other. We are both excited to find ways to improve healthcare. This past year my wife and I attended the World Health Assembly with a delegation from the World Federation of Chiropractic. In 2012, the World Health Organization published data from the Global Burden of Disease study, which looked at poor health and disability arising from all ailments in 187 countries. Low back pain was identified as the number one cause of disability worldwide. Healthcare providers, including doctors of chiropractic are addressing this serious issue. I believe it is tremendously important that patients have broader choices, particularly for musculoskeletal conditions. I am looking forward to continuing to pursue a career in clinical research. It is a very exciting field with many opportunities for young chiropractors interested in musculoskeletal epidemiology and the management of musculoskeletal conditions across large populations.

Dr. Eric J. Roseen

Research Fellow

Program for Integrative Medicine & Health Care Disparities

Department of Family Medicine

Boston Medical Center

Dowling 5 South, 1 Boston Medical Center Place

Boston, MA 02118

Chiropractic Physician

Joint Ventures Physical Therapy and Fitness

2nd Floor, 654 Beacon St.

Boston, MA 02115

Phone: (617) 536-1161 ext. 132

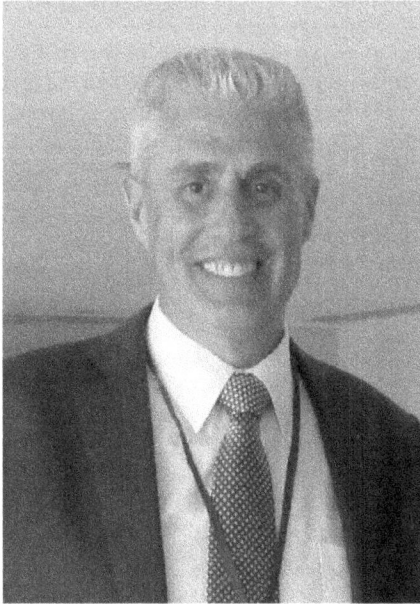

Dr. Francis X. Murphy, D.C.

"... Changed the Practices..."

In 1984 I opened a deli in Marietta Georgia, just a couple of miles from Life Chiropractic College. I was 24 years old and ready to light the world on fire with my ambition. Many of the students attending Life College were from the Northeast specifically N.J and New York. My style of deli was similar to their experience of deli's in the Northeast so they stopped by frequently, many of them were friends and acquaintances. They seemed to be another breed of health care provider, focused on the natural healing properties of the body. At the time it was all "Greek to me". Years passed and many of my friends graduated and moved on to start practicing chiropractic in other towns and cities.

One morning in April of 1988 while showering I coughed and felt a sharp pain in my back; as a 29 year old I was used to physical ailments resolving in a short time so I didn't give it a second thought. Several weeks passed and the pain in my back ebbed and intensified daily, the pain was sharp at its worse times and otherwise dull and constant. After several weeks I decided to go to a doctor and get checked out. The doctor prescribed some medicine for pain and explained I had pulled a muscle in my back. Week passed and I still had absolutely no relief from my pain. In some ways the pain had intensified and was really interfering with my breathing, sleeping and work performance. I was also becoming depressed and short tempered with my employees, friends and family.

Eventually I went to another doctor who prescribed another pain drug plus something to help me sleep. As the first treatment the drug was ineffective and the condition continued. By late summer that year I returned to the second MD for the third time, he had no alternate plan for me and suggested I see a psychologist. Feeling certain that I was mentally sound I was infuriated with the direction my health plan was taking. My depression was at a new low and I was becoming a little frightened. That day I returned to my deli feeling helpless and dejected; I had no idea what was happening to me and I couldn't see a way out of my situation. There at my deli when I arrived, sat a regular customer and student at Life Chiropractic College. I greeted him as I walked passed him and proceeded to my office where I sat in deep depression contemplating my options. Never before had I felt helpless in my life; I wanted to crawl into my head and let the world go on without me, when the customer whom I passed in the seating area at the deli requested I join him at the table for a conversation. I had no idea what was on his mind and wasn't in the mood to talk. However I agreed to speak with him, his name was Peter, and he had helped me with the construction of the deli before 1984. He got right to the point and asked me what was wrong with me. He sighted that I look badly and that my business was not running the way he was accustomed to; I could see and hear the genuine concern in his face and his voice. I told him the whole story, from the cough in the shower to the experiences with the doctors and the drugs I was taking. He listened to me with unmistakable intention to hear my story.

No sooner did I finish with that he looked me in the eye and said: "You have a rib out of place". In life sometimes you hear things for the first time that just ring true. This was one of those things. Without examining me, just listening to me Peter zeroed in on a theory that was plausible and consistent with my symptoms. I immediately inquired about the way I could address such a condition. What plan should I make to fix a rib that was out of place? He explained to me that the condition may be quite easily resolved with chiropractic adjustments. My next inquiry was the cost. The college students at Life had a price point of six dollars per visit for chiropractic care. I was shocked at the price. Immediately I was willing to give it a try. Peter gave me thorough examination. Much more detailed than any of the medical doctors had ever done to me for this problem. After the exam he carefully went over his findings with me. He was able to demonstrate to me a loss of function in one of ribs, not fully understanding at the time, Chiropractic works I inquired "What do I have to do to solve this problem? " smiled and told me that he was going to adjust my rib so that it would function properly and that the pain would subside. I asked him to adjust me right away, but out of integrity he declined stating students had to first review their findings with a staff doctor before treating patients.

I admired him for sticking to his ethics, even though I tried repeatedly to talk him into an immediate treatment. The staff doctor eventually entered the exam room. I listened while Peter reviewed his findings. He spoke with confidence and conviction about my condition and I was impressed, it wasn't long before I was lying on the adjusting table. He performed the adjustment and a loud hollow pop echoed from my thorax. The pain that had been with me seemed to drain of my body as though it were a cup of water. I took three or four deep breaths challenging the pain to reappear. It was gone!

As I drove home that afternoon it dawned on me that I knew very little about how the human body works; leading me to believe whatever anybody told me. This was a troubling thought to me. From that day on I began working toward selling my Deli and going back to School. I was going to be a Chiropractor! Graduation day was September 11th, 1995, a very proud day in my life. I was a Chiropractor!

As the years passed I flourished in my own chiropractic practice located in Dallas, Texas. I developed a thriving practice frequented by the who's who of Dallas. Over the last ten years I have been under contract with Southern Methodist University to hold a clinic on campus every Monday. I cared for over 700 athletes who participated in 17 different sports.

In May of 2006 a woman by the name of Pam Hatcher came into my practice seeking relief from the condition known as Frozen Shoulder Syndrome (FSS). This condition severely limits the range of motion of the arm at the shoulder, the pain is booth sleep inhibiting and debilitating. FSS is considered idiopathic which means it is of an unknown origin. After several weeks of treating Pam there were no results and her condition lingered on. Pam had seen many other doctors before seeking me out. She could feel my frustration with the lack of resolve for her condition, growing as time went on, and one day came to me and urged me to continue to work with her to find an answer. I agreed and dedicated myself to understanding everything I could about her condition. One evening all my research led me to a "eureka" moment; I hypothesized a cause and treatment for the condition. Miraculously the hypothesis soon led to a short resolution to her FSS. The treatment and analysis soon became a theory. The theory has undergone many tests and contains many revelations about the function of the human body. These revelations have huge implications to the Vegas nerve.

Since then, I formed a company called OtZ, which stands for One to Zero. This is a reference to on off nature of the binary system and how it relates to the on off like response the neuron system has to the OtZ adjustment. OtZ has changed the practices of

Chiropractors around the world and the lives of thousands of patients.

Whole Health Partners

6211 W NW Hwy C159

Dallas, Texas 75225

Phone: (214) 368-3030

www.wholehealthpartners.com

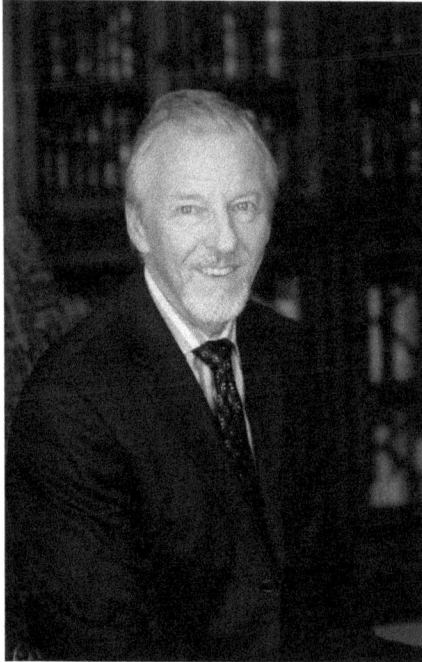

Dr. Craig Buhler, D.C.

"My Chiropractic Story"

In 1968, after trying for years to make my high school and Jr. College basketball teams, I tried out for the track team at the University of Utah as a walk on and earned an athletic scholarship. My events were the 400 meter and 1600 meter relays. Towards the end of my season, I developed pain in the top of my left foot. The training staff treated me with ice and ultrasound. I also tried different taping configurations with very little change in my pain. I also saw the team doctor who injected me with cortisone, which only lasted a day and the pain came back as soon as I started to train again. If I cut my training back, the pain was tolerable, but as soon as I started to increase my workouts, the pain came back. I laid off training for a few weeks to see if my foot would heal, but again, as soon as I started training again the pain returned.

I managed with anti-inflammatants and just pushed through the pain each season. My last season during the Western Athletic Conference Finals track meet, I ran the first heat of the time trials and scored the fastest time of my career in the fastest heat of the trials. When I finished, the pain in my foot was so severe I could hardly walk. The coach was upset because I could not compete in the relays. As a result, I lost my scholarship and dropped out of school my senior year.

I consulted an orthopedic surgeon for the ABA Utah Stars. I thought a physician for a professional basketball team would be able to figure out why my foot hurt so badly. He examined, then x-rayed my foot, and told me he could find nothing wrong with it. In frustration I told him how discouraged I was that my dream of trying out for the Olympic team would never be met. He looked at me and thought for a minute. He then said that if I was that good, he could operate and put a few screws and wires in my foot to stabilize the joint. I remember thinking how crazy that was: he could not see anything wrong and yet he wanted to do surgery. I realized that the answers to my problem did not lie in the medical field. I realized that pain was something I would have to live with.

A few years later, I was complaining to a friend that I had suffered from migraine headaches all of my life, and he suggested that I see his chiropractor. Growing up I was told by my medical doctor to avoid chiropractors, that they paralyzed people and were quacks. After voicing my concerns, my friend suggested that those comments were lies, and that I should give it a try.

My first appointment involved a full examination like I had never experienced. X-rays of my spine were taken and I was asked to schedule an appointment for a report of the findings. On the day of my next appointment our baby was sick, so we took her to the pediatrician. After our visit I asked the doctor what he thought about chiropractic, as I was to see one to review the exam and x-ray finding. His face turned red and he became angry. He commented that chiropractors were not educated enough to take x-rays, let alone read them. He went off for ten more minutes explaining how dangerous chiropractors were and that I would be crazy to see one.

I have to say, I was a little apprehensive when I walked into the chiropractors' office that day. He sat me down and explained my exam and x-ray findings and revealed the source of my headaches was coming from my neck. I had sustained an injury falling off a horse as a kid. He then took me into a treatment room and gave me my first adjustment. It was a little frightening, but when I got off the table, my headache felt better. In passing, I mentioned the old track injury and the pain I had in my foot. He laid me back down again and evaluated my foot and manipulated it. I heard a loud pop, which shocked me, but when I got off the table, I was surprised to find the pain I had experienced for five years and had cost me my dreams, was completely gone. I walked around in his office in shock. How could a problem that no one had been able to figure out be solved with one adjustment?

Over the next few months I continued to see the chiropractor for treatments for my migraines, which eventfully went away. As I sat in the waiting room waiting for my treatment I read a booklet that compared the education of a chiropractor with that of a medical doctor. I was shocked to find that chiropractic students had more in-class hours than medical students and had been a four year profession program for years. I discovered the prerequisites were the same for chiropractic students as it was for medical students. When I asked my chiropractor about it he said the requirements to become a chiropractor were just as rigid as for a medical doctor. However, chiropractic students were not required to spend time after graduation working in a hospital. I realized that my medical doctors had lied to me all those years and I realized all the opportunities I had lost because I was afraid to see a chiropractor. At that moment I realized the potential value chiropractic held for athletes struggling with injuries, and this is what I was born to do.

Once I made the decision to become a chiropractor, everything in my life began to change. It was like God took me by the shoulder and said, "Hang on young man, because this going to be a heck of a ride". Things happened in my life which led me to Western States Chiropractic College. This is where I met Dr. Alan Beardall who developed Clinical Kinesiology. His work became the basic foundation for Advanced Muscle Integration Technique or A.M.I.T.. A.M.I.T. is an integration of chiropractic and sixteen other disciplines in the healing arts and is rapidly becoming the standard of care in sports chiropractic.

After graduating from Western States Chiropractic College, I signed a contract to work for a chiropractor in Roseburg, Oregon on a preceptorship program. This allowed new graduates, who are not yet licensed, the opportunity to work with a field doctor. He had a successful practice and needed an associate. Things went well until just before Christmas. He advertised his clinic services, and at the time the Oregon Board of Chiropractic considered that unethical. They had warned him months prior but he ignored them because he felt it was his right to advertise. The Board took action and placed him on probation, and as a result my preceptorship was cancelled. My wife and I were both devastated; we were out of a job at Christmas time.

We decided to move back to Utah and got ready to take the Utah boards, in hopes of opening a clinic. I passed my boards and in May of 1998, I opened my clinic next door to a chiropractor that had been in practice for years, Dr. Hawkins. I will forever be grateful to him. Two months after opening my practice he called me and asked if I would be interested in talking with a trainer who was looking for a chiropractor to work with his basketball team. I was excited to have the opportunity to talk with a basketball trainer. It was soon after that I met Don Sparks, or "Sparky" as the players called him. The Utah Jazz has just moved from New Orleans to Salt Lake and Sparky was in the process of interviewing for team orthopedist, internist, podiatrist and physical therapist. After Sparky interviewed me, I worked on a problem he had struggled with for years. When he got off the table, he said he felt much better.

I was fortunate that during my four year chiropractic education I had the privilege of training with Dr. Alan Beardall who treated many professional athletes. This meant that when I started my practice I had an advanced skill level beyond my chiropractic training. A few days later Sparky called and asked if I would be willing to see the team's premiere forward who was struggling with lower back issues. He came in for treatment and was soon pain free.

This was the beginning of my 26 year relationship with the NBA's Utah Jazz, serving as their team chiropractor. I had the privilege of working with some of the finest athletes in the world. The Jazz training staff had the foresight to integrate the best of the medical and chiropractic fields, which resulted in the lowest games missed due to injury rates of any NBA team over a twenty year period. Over the twenty years, the Utah Jazz made it into the play-offs 19 times, won the Mid-West Division Championship six times, and won the Western Conference Championship twice to move on to the NBA Finals against the Chicago Bulls and Michael Jordan.

Over my 38 year career I have worked with thousands of broken down athletes, many who were ready to give up their sport and their dreams of making a high school, college, or professional team. Many have aspired to make the Olympic team. After lengthy therapy, they all made the team. Many of those who made the Olympic team went on to win bronze, silver and gold medals for the United States or Australia.

My professional journey has often been met with violent opposition by the medical community but has also been filled with appreciation from my patients who realized their dreams. During John Stockton's acceptance speech into the NBA Hall of Fame, he gave me credit for helping him extend his career.

I love this profession and the lives it has allowed me to touch. I recognize that I have been able to stand on the shoulders of great chiropractic physicians who I consider "healers" which helped me get to where I am today. My vision is that chiropractic and Advanced Muscle Integration Techniques will soon become the standard of care for sports related injuries and the future of health care.

Craig F. Buhler, D.C., F.I.C.C.

447 N. 300 W. #5

Kaysville, Utah, 84037

www.amitmethod.com

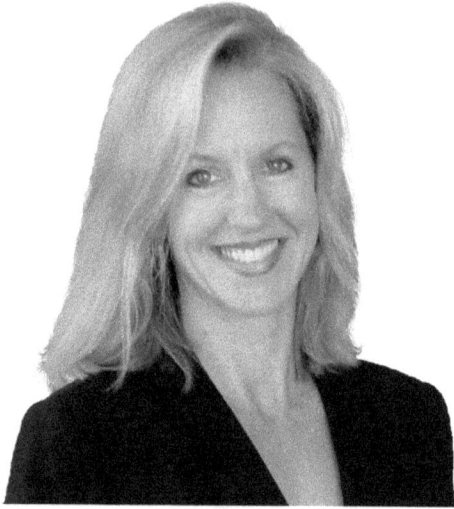

Dr. Kelli Pearson

D.C., D.A.B.C.O., F.I.C.C.

"Paying It Forward..."

I grew up with my mom telling me that anything was possible, and a father who strongly encouraged me to do the right thing. As a youngster, I was drawn to those bound to a wheelchair or affected by some type of health challenge. Though not understanding my urge to reach out, it became clear I wanted to help, through touch.

Fast forward to my time at UCLA many years later. Kinesiology seemed a good major, as I prepared for some sort of healing profession. I resisted approaches that required only minimal physical contact, writing scripts or talk therapy, and was not fond of scalpels and blood, particularly if it involved working on those who were not in a condition to talk back.

Assuming good grades would be necessary for success, in addition to the postgraduate studies needed, I graduated as Salutatorian in the College of Bachelors and Science. However, my frustration mounted by my Junior year, as I was still confused about my next steps. Just months away from graduation, I applied to the Physical Therapy pro-gram at San Francisco State University and was accepted. UCLA had a rehab hospital, so I headed off to observe there. Instead of experiencing an atmosphere of hope and excitement, a day at the ward left me depressed; I was certain that this was not my calling. Most of the patients were either victims of motorcycle accidents with brain injuries or amputees. While improvement and rehabilitation were certainly possible for these folks, the path involved was too slow for my temperament.

Graduation was looming, with still no direction. Westwood, the home of UCLA, had many alternative opportunities for learning. At the end of my senior year, I enrolled in the Los Angeles School of Massage. At that time, only 100 hours were required for graduation, in contrast to the 500 plus needed today. It was evident to me that this profession would demand more rigorous training to become truly competent, but I completed it, nonetheless and gained tools in therapeutic touch that would prove to be useful in the long run.

Down the street from my apartment was a premier school of Jin Shin Do, run by Iona and Ron Teegarden. Iona still teaches today and is considered one of the' outstanding practitioners in this field. I launched into this training of acupressure. The art of using fingertip pressure along the meridians to support healing allowed me to gain respect for the power of moving energy or chi. At the end of this training, I felt one step closer to finding my way, but this work seemed too slow and the results a bit too intangible. I felt intuitive that there was a profession that would allow me to touch people and see measurable changes more quickly. As I look back now, my impatience served me well in my pursuit!

Graduation had come and gone, and my father was now showing concern. The checks to supplement my room and the board had stopped coming as it was my turn to support myself. I worked as a waitress in an upscale steak house. Wealthy clientele and their tips kept me afloat, but I was treading water. My father offered to pay for medical school. This incredibly generous offer looked tempting, but I knew it was the wrong path for me. Orthodox medicine was not my passion. There had to be a better healing path for me than writing scripts for medication.

An unexpected event that happened next was nothing short of a miracle. One sunny afternoon, while standing at a crosswalk waiting for the traffic light to change, my eyes were drawn to a very tall man standing to my left. He was at least six feet tall, but with his Sikh turban; he looked seven feet tall. A Caucasian Sikh was not a unique site in Santa Monica, but somehow his unusual presence caught my attention. I looked up to the left and caught his smile. He only said, "Do you want to come and watch me where I work?" Dumbfounded, to my surprise, I quickly said "Yes," and we walked in silence for three blocks to his office. One would think that a few more questions might have been appropriate before I blindly following a stranger to an unknown destiny, but on that day, it seemed like the right thing to do, to follow along in silence and without question.

When we approached his office, I did not bother to study the writing on the door or look for a sign. Instead, we walked in, to find a man perched uncomfortably on a chair in the reception area. My new friend asked him to come down the hall, signaling me to follow. I observed as he listened compassionately to this gentleman's story about how he ended up bent over and in pain. The Sikh then moved him around on the examination table, exploring his limitations. What happened next took me by surprise. It seemed to my untrained eye that he pounced on this man, followed by a great cracking sound emanating from his lower back. The man got off the table much quicker than when he got on, this time with a smile on his face and standing much straighter.

I had a sense of excitement as we walked towards the reception to find his next patient. This time, a woman was holding her head in her hands. When the Sikh asked her to follow him back, it was evident she had been crying. Still, no words had been exchanged between this mystery man and myself. He guided her back to the room with a hand on her shoulder, turned down the lights, and began listening to her story. As he had done for the gentleman before, after a period of listening, he carefully started moving her neck and shoulders and feeling her spine. While gently holding her head one moment, he asked her to breathe and with lightning speed, moved her head to the right, and another great crack resounded, this time emanating from her neck. She instantly began to cry, and my heart sank. I felt that perhaps the expectation of success with this method was too good to be true. But then, I realized she was crying with happiness as she informed him her headache was finally gone.

Walking back down the hall, I tapped him on the shoulder. "What are you?" Up to that point, I had never had any interaction with a Chiropractor, having heard that they were quacks. He smiled and explained he was a Chiropractor, and he was restoring the natural ability of his patients to heal. He then encouraged me to attend a spinal care class that evening. Sitting in that room, I finally realized without a shadow of a doubt, that I had found my calling. The next step was to go about planning for my education.

I loved the West Coast but wanted out of the Los Angeles area. I learned of a new Chiropractic College in Sunnyvale, near the city of San Jose, called Northern California College of Chiropractic. Residing close to my hometown, I matriculated at my first opportunity. My commitment to the right grades at UCLA made this an easy accomplishment. Since the school was so new, the college had not yet been recognized by the Council on Chiropractic Education, and would take some time. Despite that, I know it would only be a matter of time, and I was right to have chosen to study there.

Having no money at the time did not deter me. I found two jobs, one teaching exercise classes at a nearby gym, and one waiting tables at another excellent restaurant. Thankfully, the college did manage to achieve accreditation late in my studies, which allowed me to secure a $5,000 loan, tiny by comparison to the student debt today.

The moment I sat down in the chair that first day at school, I felt at home. My father was concerned that his daughter would throw her life away pursuing such a poorly understood discipline. However, his upset was soon set aside after he developed acute lower back pain, and was unable to find a cure through allopathic medicine. After much distress, he traveled down to the college where I had my good friend and mentor, Dr. Ed Cremata, care for him and resolve his condition. Ed was not yet graduated, but his commitment to chiropractic and his skill set helped my dad immediately feel much better. To this day, my dad still gets regular chiropractic care. My heartfelt thanks go out to Dr. Cremata, who continues to do amazing work today, for that critical and strategic success!

Since that magical day long ago when I met my 7 foot tall Chiropractic friend, his identity and location have remained a mystery to me, in spite of my attempts to locate him. I hope that this book somehow ends up in his hands one day so that he will know of my eternal gratitude for taking that chance to reach out to me way back when on that sunny day in Los Angeles. In turn, my husband, Dr. Dana Weary and I have trained several young people over our 30 plus years in practice, as we try to honor those who paved the way for us. As our younger doctors grow to become successful in their careers and healing abilities, we feel grateful for the opportunity to "pay it forward" and invest in the future of this wonderful profession!

Pearson & Weary Pain Relief Clinic

N 1410 Mullan Ste 200

Spokane, WA 99206

Phone: (509) 927-8997

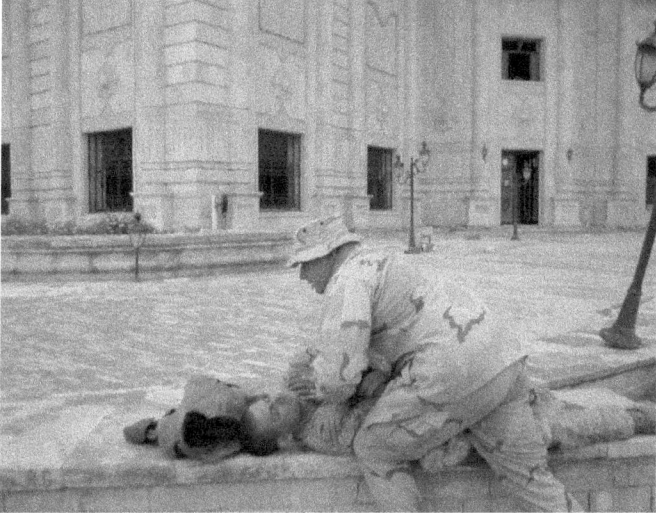

Dr. Mark Losack

D.C., CCSP®, F.I.C.C.

Colonel USMC (Retired)

"...Sincere Appreciation..."

I was introduced to Chiropractic in 1976, during my undergraduate years at Lamar University. I was watching CBS 60 Minutes and they did a story on Chiropractors and the changes in the profession. Dr. Leroy Perry was featured as was Dr. Sid Williams. Dwight Stone, the world record holder in the high jump was featured and talked about the athletes bringing their own Chiropractors to care for them at the Olympic Games because the medical officials at the US Olympic Committee did not recognize Chiropractors as necessary. I thought about visiting a Chiropractor but did not because I was told the treatment would cost nine dollars and who had nine dollars lying around?

As a young Marine officer returning from Operation Desert Shield/Desert Storm, I knew that I was ready for a new beginning. I was stationed in Hawaii and was truly in paradise. I wanted to stay in Hawaii, so I began making plans to attend University of Hawaii medical school.

I was dating a woman who lived in Pasadena, California. During a visit to her home my neck stiffened to a point that I was unable to check the side view mirrors while driving without twisting my whole body around. Truth be told, I developed the nervous habit of "cracking" my neck while I deployed and had over torqued it while visiting her.

For some reason I asked if she or her mom knew a Chiropractor. They recommended Dr. Michael Budincich. As Dr. "Bud" was treating me, I began thinking "I wonder what it takes to be a Chiropractor?" I received his new patient packet which contained information about Chiropractic, how it's about natural healing, the importance of the nervous system and the spine, and how that relationship affects one's health. It also had the phone number for the Council on Chiropractic Education.

As my girlfriend and I were driving away, I asked what she thought of me looking into becoming a Chiropractor. She laughed and said, "When I saw you and Dr. Bud walking out together, I thought, Mark would be a good Chiropractor.''

I called the CCE and they sent materials about the profession. I focused on two schools; one in my home state of Texas and one in the Whittier, California. At the end of the day, I decided to stay in California for school and for the girl.

Entering school, I was oblivious to the challenges Chiropractors were facing. I had no idea that the American Medical Association had tried and failed to eradicate the profession of Chiropractic or that they considered it unethical for medical doctors to associate with Chiropractors. In the early years of the profession, some Chiropractors had been jailed on trumped up charges of practicing medicine without a license.

As I began my Chiropractic education, I became aware of rifts within the profession itself, that at times, were more damaging than attacks from the outside. I observed that as growing research supported the effectiveness of Chiropractic care for low back and eventually neck pain, that other providers, e.g., physical therapists, began practicing spinal manipulation, which, by and large they had not done in the past. It appeared to be the theme of the era; somebody has an effective solution and others co-opt the idea or method as their own.

During Chiropractic college, I saw the importance, indeed the professional responsibility, of being a member of a professional association. I became involved with the Student American Chiropractic Association where I served as a class representative and eventually the President of the Los Angeles College of Chiropractic chapter.

After graduation, I established my practice in Oceanside, California, near San Diego. By this time my girlfriend had become my wife and we had a one year old son, with another son soon to follow.

I volunteered to work with Oceanside High School's sports medicine team and for some years was the only doctor on the sidelines. I enjoyed working with the athletes and established a reputation with the coaches for keeping players in the game. The athletic trainer and I worked closely together building trust and friendship.

My practice was steadily increasing to a point that I was looking for a larger facility. Then 9/11 happened. I had remained in the Marine Corps Reserve after Desert Storm. In October of 2002, I was informed that I was being recalled to active duty in two weeks. I was able to refer my patients to three other doctors, thinking that when I returned some would return to me and others would remain with the new doctors.

I deployed in January 2003 on board the USS Boxer bound for Iraq. While on board, I began treating many Marines and Sailors. At one point I was asked by a Medical Officer to treat some of the Marines in his infantry battalion. He had done all he could and was out of options for them. I treated the Marines everyday for two weeks; sometimes adjusting them three times per day.

I was assigned to 1st Marine Division and eventually found myself with the Forward Combat Operations Center. This element became Task Force Tripoli and seized Saddam's hometown of Tikrit. I continued to treat Marines and Sailors during lulls in combat operations. Our task force turned Tikrit over to the US Army's 4th Infantry Division and we returned south. I was reassigned to I Marine Expeditionary Force. As I was unloading my gear in the I MEF headquarters area, a junior officer walked by and asked if I was a Chiropractor. I replied that I was. Most of the personnel assigned to this headquarters knew I was a Chiropractor and that question was often followed by "Sir I'm having a problem and wondered if you could adjust me." This time the junior officer followed with "Sir you have to stop that. I just got off the phone with Headquarters Marine Corps and the Navy's Bureau of Medicine said that some Marine named Losack was providing Chiropractic care to the troops and needed to stop." I informed the younger officer, that I had no intention of stopping. BUMED had no command authority, neither did Headquarters Marine Corps. I told him that I had taken an oath to provide care and that I could no more stop adjusting those that needed it than he could live without breathing. He said, "Ok sir, but just letting you know that they are out to get you."

I returned home in June of 2003. After several months of decompressing, I took steps to renew my practice. No sooner had I began the practice part time than I MEF began plans to return to Iraq and relieve the 82d Airborne Division in Al Anbar province. For the second time I shut down my practice and deployed to Iraq again. During the first battle of Fallujah, I realized two things. First, the need for Marine officers with my skill set was not going away. Second, I could not sustain starting and stopping my practice. With that I requested to remain on active duty. From 2004 through 2009 I continued to serve as a Marine Colonel in various capacities in combat and humanitarian operations across the globe. During this time, I continued to provide Chiropractic care to anyone who asked. Once another officer approached me about providing care for his father who was visiting him and had a back issue. The smiles on their faces after care tells the whole story.

In 2009, I retired from the Marine Corps and began teaching at the Los Angeles College of Chiropractic. It was good to be back at my alma mater and back in Chiropractic. I wanted to instill in my students the sacred trust that was being handed to them as the future of the Chiropractic. I returned to full time private practice in June of 2013.

Of all my experiences since choosing to become a Chiropractor, I can think of none more fulfilling than ending the practice day, exhausted from facilitating patient's rapid recovery and them expressing their sincere appreciation by referring friends and family for care.

Dr. Mark Losack

Oceanside Chiropractic and Sports Medicine

Email: dr.losack@gmail.com

Phone: 619-990-5594

... and the Institutions

Leading the Way

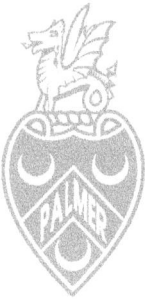

PALMER
College of Chiropractic

Palmer College of Chiropractic

"The Legacy and Leadership…"

The Legacy and Leadership of Palmer College of Chiropractic

As the first and largest chiropractic college in the world, Palmer College of Chiropractic leads the way for the growth of the profession and chiropractic education. Since its founding in 1897 by the discoverer of chiropractic, D.D. Palmer, it has sent nearly 50,000 alumni out to practice worldwide – one-third of all chiropractors in the United States are Palmer College graduates.

Palmer College of Chiropractic is known as *The* Trusted Leader in Chiropractic Education®, and has set forth an identity for chiropractors as the primary care professionals for spinal health and well-being.

Science and technology blend with rich tradition at Palmer. Just as D.D. Palmer blazed the first path toward a chiropractic profession, the three Palmer campuses today are charting new territory in contemporary chiropractic education through innovations in student learning, patient care and research. The main campus is in Davenport, Iowa, where D.D. Palmer performed the first chiropractic adjustment in 1895. The two branch campuses are in San Jose, Calif., and Port Orange, Fla.

Research leadership

From its inception, Palmer College has been a leader with vision that continues to embrace the pioneering spirit of its founder. One example is the Palmer Center for Chiropractic Research (PCCR) -- the largest research center in the world dedicated to chiropractic.

The PCCR's annual budget is approximately $5 million -- the biggest in chiropractic education. Since 1995, Palmer has received more than $35 million in grants from sources like the National Institutes of Health, the U.S. Health Resources and Services Administration and the Department of Defense.

Palmer College is the first chiropractic college to pursue translational research (research that's translated into practical applications) and the first to be awarded federal funding to implement it.

Students throughout the world come to Palmer College's three campuses because they want to learn from the leader in chiropractic education. Regardless of background, students at Palmer College all share the same goal: to become the primary care professionals for spinal health and well-being.

Through immersion in the Palmer learning environment, students experience a profound personal and professional transformation. Exposure to a wide range of hands-on, real-world care-giving experiences helps Palmer students gain skills and expand their understanding of the chiropractic profession's character of compassion, purpose and service to community.

World-renowned faculty

Palmer's learning community is anchored by its world-class faculty. Professors are keenly focused on student success and producing exceptional doctors of chiropractic. Palmer College's educators are highly regarded scholars, many of whom continue to work in chiropractic practices and share their real-world experiences in the classroom. With a student-to-faculty ratio of 15:1 or better, faculty get to know their students well and readily provide one-on-one attention within a welcoming open-door atmosphere. Among Palmer College's forward-thinking faculty and administrators are distinguished speakers, researchers and authors who've written textbooks used in many chiropractic colleges and who help lead the chiropractic profession.

Largest network of clinics

The Palmer Chiropractic Clinics -- a network of outpatient and community outreach clinics in the three campus communities -- make up the largest clinic system in chiropractic education. During Palmer's 2013-14 fiscal year there were a total of 147,672 patient visits to Palmer Chiropractic Clinics in Davenport, Iowa; Moline, Ill.; San Jose, Calif.; and Port Orange, Fla. Nearly 12,800 of those visits were by active-duty military members and their families, as well as disabled veterans. These patients received complimentary care from Palmer in gratitude for their military service.

Students have a number of options to gain hands-on clinical experience with patients. In addition to caring for patients under the supervision of faculty mentors in the clinic system, students may serve preceptorships with practicing chiropractors throughout the country during their last term. Or they can participate in military health-care internships and work alongside a practicing doctor in a Veterans Health Administration or military hospital setting.

Focus on student success

Student success, before and after graduation, is paramount at Palmer. The Palmer Center for Business Development offers free business programs and services for students and alumni – plus an online career networking placement service. In any given month on the Palmer CareerNetwork there are up to 1,300 associate positions available or practices for sale. The College also offers a program to help students reduce their debt load while in school and plan for their financial well-being after graduation. And each year, more than $2.5 million in scholarships is awarded to students.

These efforts are paying dividends. Palmer's 2011 student-loan default rate for its students is extremely low at 3.3 percent; the 2012 draft rate of 2.4 percent (official rate expected in September 2015) is even lower. Compare this to the average student-loan default rate for chiropractic college students at 7 percent, and the average for all U.S. college students at 13.7 percent.

An April 2015 study by the prestigious Brookings Institution lists Palmer in the top colleges with respect to college-loan repayment with a perfect score of 100. Brookings also gave Palmer a score of 99 for occupational earnings power -- a measure that expresses the average market value of the career for which the college prepared its graduates. According to a May 2015 article in MarketWatch.com, Palmer is No. 4 among U.S. colleges for student-loan repayment.

In short, Palmer earns its reputation as *The* Trusted Leader in Chiropractic Education in a myriad of ways. The overarching goal of Palmer College of Chiropractic is to educate the finest doctors of chiropractic who are well prepared for both patient care and business aspects of contemporary chiropractic practice.

One college with three campuses

Each Palmer campus offers students the same high-quality, experience-based education, but with unique regional, recreational or cultural activities.

Davenport, Iowa, Campus:

Davenport, Iowa, is where chiropractic was born. D.D. Palmer performed the first chiropractic adjustment in 1895 and founded Palmer College of Chiropractic in the heart of Davenport, within blocks of the Mississippi River. Davenport is part of a larger metropolitan area of 400,000 known as the Quad Cities. With two Palmer outpatient clinics plus two community outreach clinics that provide care to underserved patients, senior Palmer students have ample opportunities to work directly with patients. From athletic teams to intramurals to club sports, Palmer students find various ways to keep fit and stay active. Community participation is also an important part of the Palmer experience. During the world-famous Bix 7 Road Race -- one of many events staffed by Palmer students -- Sports Council members offer hands-on care to athletes.

Port Orange, Florida, Campus:

The Port Orange, Fla., campus opened in 2002. It's located just minutes from Daytona Beach and about an hour northeast of Orlando. Port Orange (pop. 57,203) is a quiet and affordable neighborhood community. The vibrant greater metropolitan area, with a population of 2.5 million and nearby lakes and beaches offer students a wide range of entertainment and recreational activities. Senior-level students master their clinical skills in the Palmer outpatient clinic as well as a community outreach clinic. Palmer Sports Council students work directly with athletes in numerous events, including the Ragnar Relay in the Florida Keys and the Nautica USLA National Lifeguard Championships.

San Jose, California, Campus:

The San Jose, Calif., campus, established in 1980, is located in the hub of world-renowned Silicon Valley. Living in one of the safest cities per capita in the country, Palmer students have easy access to multicultural San Jose (pop. 998,789) and nearby beaches and mountains. Senior students gain experience in the on-campus Palmer Chiropractic Clinic as well as in a network of community outreach clinics that care for underserved patients. As part of one of the largest and most active Sports Council groups in chiropractic education, Sports Council members offer care at numerous high-profile sporting events throughout the year, including the world's premier cycling festival, the Sea Otter Classic, in Monterey, Calif., and the Silicon Valley Turkey Trot Thanksgiving Day 5K community fundraiser in San Jose.

Davenport, Iowa, Campus:

1000 Brady St., Davenport, IA 52803

1 (800) 722-3648

admissions.ia@palmer.edu

Port Orange, Florida, Campus:

4777 City Center Parkway

Port Orange, FL 32129

1 (866) 585-9677

admissions.fl@palmer.edu

San Jose, California, Campus:

90 E. Tasman Dr.

San Jose, CA 95134

1 (866) 303-7939

admissions.ca@palmer.edu

www.palmer.edu

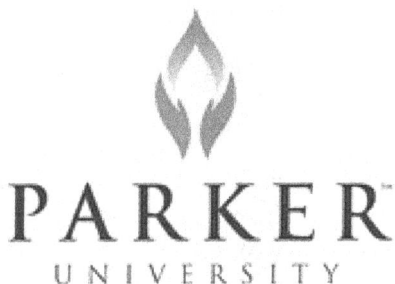

PARKER
UNIVERSITY

Parker University

"For more than Three Decades..."

For more than three decades, Parker University has provided exemplary chiropractic education that offers excellent training in both clinical practice and business expertise. The overarching emphasis of these critical components of the curriculum is the development of the compassion to serve our fellow human beings drawn from the teachings of Dr. James W. Parker.

Parker University (formerly Parker College of Chiropractic) is named for its late founder, Dr. James William Parker. After a successful career as a chiropractor and the founder of the world famous Parker Seminars in 1951, Dr. Parker helped establish and fund Parker College of Chiropractic in 1982. Dr. Parker imbued the new institution with a unique combination of healing, philosophy and business training. The nontraditional approach to chiropractic education became the cornerstone for Parker College and continues to inform the Parker University of today.

In April, 2011 Parker College of Chiropractic officially became Parker University. In addition to the College of Chiropractic, Parker University now has the College of Business and Technology and the College of Health Sciences. These new colleges offer programs in Radiologic Technology, Occupational Therapy Assistant, Massage Therapy, Computer Information Science, Masters in Business Administration and many others both on line and on campus.

The MBA is designed for self-employed chiropractors who want to improve and expand their practices or open multiple facilities. The program may be completed online to best serve the needs of doctors in practice. These programs will equip professionals with the skills to thrive in these growing career paths and help change the health care paradigm in the United States to one focused on wellness.

All of these new programs add to the rich tradition of innovative and leading edge education for professionals in healthcare and related occupational paths. These innovations are being further developed by Dr. Brian McAulay who became president of Parker in 2013. Under Dr. McAulay's leadership the university is exploring further academic developments and is taking a leadership role in the nurturance of productive partnerships in Dallas/Ft. Worth, the region, the nation and internationally.

WHY CHOOSE PARKER UNIVERSITY?

Parker has more than one thousand students currently enrolled. The university is expected to grow to approximately two thousand five hundred students by 2020. The university is reaching out to new populations and communicating with young people who have a strong interest in the natural, holistic approaches to total wellbeing. Strong students who respect the healing power of the body and who have the passion to create their own success while improving the lives of others are the right fit for Parker University.

Parker's educational philosophy is encapsulated in one of the Parker Principles created by the founder, Dr. James Parker – Loving service is my first technique. Finding a profession that allows loving service to be foremost is the path toward a lifetime of fulfillment for those who want to make a difference in the world. That is what the chiropractic calling provides. Parker University has the curriculum, the faculty and the facilities that are second to none in chiropractic education. Our graduates devote their professional lives to giving their patients the loving service that is the hallmark of chiropractic care.

Our students have the advantage of facilities that are the best in chiropractic. Our classrooms have the latest teaching technology and the Gross Anatomy Laboratory is the envy of the chiropractic world. The Parker Wellness Clinic is a 30,000 square foot facility where our student interns perfect the art of chiropractic care under the supervision of the best chiropractor/mentors in the profession.

An excellent example of the commitment to the latest in teaching technology is the acquisition of the Force Sensing Table Technology (FSTT) made possible by the generosity of Dr. John and Niki Dealey of Dallas. Dr. Dealey is a member of the Parker Board of Trustees. The FSTT uses force sensing tables contained in a mannequin that provide immediate data on the speed and strength of manual techniques employed by chiropractic students during training. This device will be one of the few in the United States and will allow the student and professor feedback on performance of the adjustment technique being applied.

The enrollment in the College of Chiropractic is approximately

750 students. Large enough for a remarkable diversity of student backgrounds and experiences but small enough that the individual student remains the single most important feature of the ten trimester academic program.

During the three year and four month program our students are exposed to an educational exercise that is challenging and exhilarating. It prepares them for the lifelong learning that is part of chiropractic practice. The emphasis on business readiness makes them uniquely prepared to become independent leaders in their communities and in the practice of their healing art.

VISIT THE PARKER CAMPUS

Prospective students are strongly encouraged to visit our Dallas campus. Parker Power Weekends are an especially good opportunity to learn more about the course of study and the supportive, family-like environment of the university. Visit our web site www.parker.edu or call 800-637-8337 for more information on the university and opportunities to visit.

Parker University

2540 Walnut Hill Lane

Dallas, TX 75229

Phone: (800) 637-8337

Email: future@parker.edu

www.parker.edu

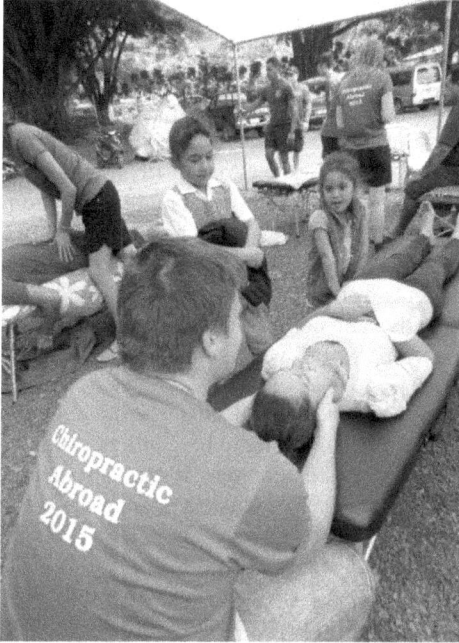

The New Zealand College of Chiropractic

"New Zealand's Best Kept Secret..."

In 1979, the New Zealand Royal Commission of Inquiry released its report on chiropractic. This report endorsed chiropractic as part of New Zealand's healthcare system, and one of its many recommendations was to establish chiropractic education in New Zealand. This report, in combination with a very dedicated group of chiropractors, was the catalyst to open a chiropractic college. Up until the College opened, New Zealanders travelled overseas to study chiropractic.

In 1994, the College opened under the governance of the New Zealand Chiropractors' Association. In 1999, ownership was transferred to the New Zealand Chiropractic Education Trust Board and the College was renamed the New Zealand College of Chiropractic. Today, the College is a world-renowned institution attracting students from all over the world, producing world-leading, innovative and cutting edge chiropractic research and is a global leader with a world-wide reputation for excellence.

The College attracts amazing students who are committed to their studies and have a strong desire to help others. Although the College has the highest requirement of any chiropractic college in the world, 96% of students graduate and enter the profession and practice around the world.

The commitment to excellence extends to not only the curriculum, faculty and staff but also to The Centre for Chiropractic Research. Located at the College, it is a world-leading research centre producing ground-breaking chiropractic research. The key focus for the researchers is to explore how chiropractic care helps restore dysfunctional central nerve system processes and how chiropractic care prevents problems from happening in the first place. The research team is the link in the delivery of the philosophy, science and art of chiropractic. The sweet spot for the New Zealand College of Chiropractic is the ability to bring the science through research to the philosophy and art of chiropractic.

Since 2008, the New Zealand Chiropractic Board, the New Zealand Chiropractors' Association and the New Zealand Chiropractic Education Trust Board have worked together under a memorandum of understanding and together they represent and govern the New Zealand chiropractic profession.

The College is a small boutique institution with no more than 300 students which includes approximately 100 international students. The College graduates around 75 students each year.

The growing reputation of the College means that each year, there are more applications received than places available. The College admissions processes ensure each student is motivated and is able to meet the study demands of the curriculum. It accounts for the high completion rate and mirrors the mission statement of the College – educating great people to become the world's best chiropractors.

As a result of a comprehensive admissions process, the College attracts only the very best chiropractic students. Students regularly win awards, competitions and scholarships. Students have won the Independent Tertiary Education New Zealand awards for the last two years. Currently, the Talk the Tic world champion is a 2nd year student, who competed against students from chiropractic colleges from around the world. Students are active and prominent members of the World Congress of Chiropractic Students (WCCS), and the 3rd year students participate in an annual outreach community service program in Rarotonga at their own cost. All students are involved in research, and in collaboration with lecturers, a growing number of students are publishing journal articles.

The College is known as the 'small giant' of chiropractic education providers globally. Although relatively small, the College is recognized as one of the best in the world and slowly this best kept secret is not so secret anymore.

New Zealand College of Chiropractic

PO Box 113-044

Newmarket

Auckland 1149

New Zealand

Phone: +64 9 526 6789

Fax: +64 9 526 6788

www.chiropractic.ac.nz

www.ingramcontent.com/pod-product-compliance
Lightning Source LLC
Chambersburg PA
CBHW072249270326
41930CB00010B/2317